THE
EXERCISE
BALL Bible

Over 200 exercises to help you lose
weight and improve your fitness,
strength, flexibility and posture

LUCY KNIGHT

KYLE BOOKS

First published in Great Britain in 2012 by
Kyle Books
23 Howland Street
London W1T 4AY
general.enquiries@kylebooks.com
www.kylebooks.com

ISBN: 978-0-85783-022-7

Text © 2012 Lucy Knight
Photography © 2012 Tony Chau
Design © 2012 Kyle Books

Editor: Catharine Robertson
Designer: Heidi Baker
Photographer: Tony Chau
Copy editor: Barbara Archer
Indexer: Helen Snaith
Models: Delphine Gaborit, Chris Willis, Jemma Walker, Ethan Palczynski, Lisa Curwen
Hair and make-up: Alisha Bailey, Katy Nixon, Marie Coulter, Beth Margetts
Production: Nic Jones and Gemma John

A Cataloguing In Publication record for this title is available from the British Library.

Printed and bound in China by Toppan Leefung Printing Ltd.

DISCLAIMER: The author and publisher cannot accept any responsibility for misadventure resulting from the practice of any of the exercises in this book. It is not intended and should not be used as guidance for the treatment of serious health problems; please refer to a medical professional if you have concerns about any aspect of your condition or fitness level.

CONTENTS

INTRODUCTION   6

CHAPTER ONE : GETTING STARTED   10

CHAPTER TWO : TONING AND STRENGTHENING   50
                     WITH THE BALL

CHAPTER THREE : AEROBICS WITH THE BALL   94

CHAPTER FOUR : PILATES WITH THE BALL   126

CHAPTER FIVE : YOGA WITH THE BALL   158

CHAPTER SIX : BALL STRETCHES   194

CHAPTER SEVEN : HEALTHY BACK AND POSTURE   218

CHAPTER EIGHT : PREGNANCY, BIRTHING   238
                 AND BEYOND

CHAPTER NINE : DE-STRESS WITH THE BALL   268

RESOURCES   284

INDEX   285

INTRODUCTION

Exercise balls are taking over the world! There are people rolling around on them in every health and fitness centre, ball classes are appearing on every studio's timetable and interestingly, more and more people have one in their home. Unfortunately some people still haven't realised the full potential of the rubber orb they have stashed away in their cupboard; it really is undoubtedly one of the most useful and versatile pieces of exercise equipment you could own.

This book is intended as a comprehensive guide to the many different ways in which you can make use of your ball, and offers a workout option for your every mood and stage of life. This amazing piece of rubber, as well as being an exercise option in its own right, can also add an element of interest and challenge to many other workout forms, such as yoga and Pilates. For many women it is even becoming part of their antenatal routine as well as their birthing partner of choice.

By reading this book I would like you to embark on a whole new curious relationship with your exercise ball, one in which this comfortable ball of rubber can become your support, both physically and psychologically, enabling you to achieve your goals. The ball can be used to support your weight when things are difficult and to challenge your balance and range of movement when you feel ready. Use the ball to create a fantastically fun, high-energy aerobics session, followed by something to deliciously stretch around and meditate on.

I am sure that by the end of this book you will, like me, feel quite attached to your new circular friend and will be amazed by the limitless options it provides.

A SHORT HISTORY

The ball was invented in 1963 by Aquilino Cosani, an Italian toy-maker, and was called the Gymnastik. Since then it has had many names, including Swiss, physio, flexi, gym and exercise ball to name a few. Shortly after its invention, the ball was seen being used in physiotherapy circles in Switzerland – hence 'Swiss ball'. It was first used by an English physiotherapist, Mary Quinton, who incorporated it into her programmes for children with cerebral palsy.

In the late 1960s Dr Susan Klein-Vogelbach, the founding director of a Swiss physiotherapy school, started to use the ball in adult orthopaedic therapies, back rehabilitation and postural realignment. By the 1980s, visiting American physical therapists had discovered the ball and brought the knowledge back to the US. It was during the early 1990s that the exercise ball moved from rehabilitation settings into the fitness arena, becoming a big part of the core strengthening trend that was gathering pace.

Over the past decade there has been a significant increase in the use of stability ball workouts in mainstream gyms and health and fitness centres. It is recognised as an adaptable exercise tool for people of all ages and abilities to enhance their exercise programme and other areas of life.

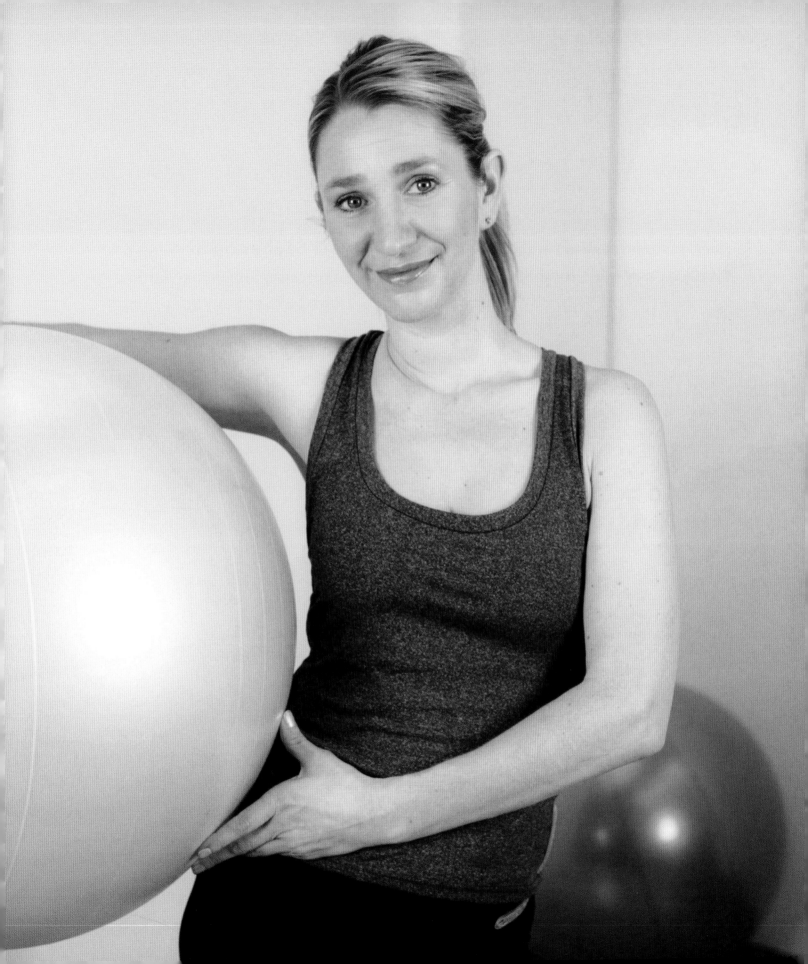

BALL BENEFITS

First, exercise balls are cheap. They can be bought from a variety of large stores or websites for less than the price of an exercise class. Once you have one, it is very easy to store without taking up the whole of your spare room.

What makes the ball unique, though, are the benefits that come about from exercising on a round surface. This gives you a much greater range of movement than a flat surface such as the floor, meaning you get your body into positions that would otherwise be impossible, allowing you to stretch, strengthen and isolate every muscle – some you never realised existed.

Its roundness also means you are exercising on an unstable base of support, therefore anything you decide to do on it requires balance, balance, balance! The body, when faced with this challenge, recruits deep stabilising muscles, many of which are otherwise often neglected, resulting in common injuries of the knees, ankles, shoulders and back. It is also the strengthening of these muscles that aids greatly in the prevention of more debilitating back problems that cost industry millions each year. An estimated 7–10 million of us suffer from back problems. All a reminder of our increasingly sedentary lifestyles and working environments; too many hours slouched over our computer or sat in front of our favourite TV 'soap'.

You will also notice that just sitting on the ball demands good posture. In fact, if you slouch on the ball in the same way you do on your sofa, you will simply fall off! Good posture once practised on the ball will be carried into the rest of your life with huge benefits, not only in terms of injury prevention but also in terms of your appearance and confidence. This is explored in greater detail in Chapter 7.

The ball is also a master at providing functional movement skills. Functional movement means exactly that: training your body to be able to perform the everyday tasks and movement needed to function in everyday life. For example, staying strong, flexible and confident enough to engage in fun and adventurous activities with your children, without the fear of putting your back out when throwing them into the air!

Using an exercise ball can also help you to stay mobile in later life. This could be the key to living out your retirement the way you have always hoped, with full independence, as opposed to feeling trapped in your home or having to rely on others. Loss of strength and flexibility occurs naturally as part of the ageing process and yet simple regular exercise with the ball can make a massive difference, reducing the impact this would otherwise have on your quality of life. Functional movement is the chance to practise everyday movements that some of us take for granted, ensuring that these abilities stay with us for years to come.

The ball can add interest to your regular fitness regime by opening up a whole new repertoire of exercise options right across the spectrum. Pilates instructors are able to recreate some of the exercises normally executed on expensive, specialised reformer equipment as well as add an extra challenge to matwork exercises. This is discussed further in Chapter 4.

In yoga, by introducing the ball into your practice you will add an entirely new dimension to your workouts. You will find you are able to get your body into postures otherwise impossible and add an extra balance challenge along the way! Chapter 5 discusses this further.

If your goal is to tone up, the exercise options are endless and much more fun with a ball in tow. You can even use your ball as a comfortable bench for those dumbbell exercises usually seen in the gym, with the added benefit of simultaneously working your core muscles to keep you steady on the ball. This is discussed further in Chapter 2.

If fat burning or weight loss is your aim, then the ball can deliver a dynamic yet safe cardiovascular workout and I can guarantee you will not have laughed as much in any other aerobics-style class! Many traditional aerobics exercises can be adapted to the ball as well as using it to throw and catch, bounce up and down on and create a whole array of circling and lifting choreography. The ball absorbs some of the impact normally associated with high impact aerobic exercise, making it a much kinder option for your joints. This is discussed further in Chapter 3.

The benefits don't stop there. The ball is also being used more and more in antenatal classes to encourage a healthy pregnancy, assist with an active birth by shortening labour and by giving women a comfortable way of getting into appropriate birthing positions. Once the baby has arrived, it can provide a quick and enjoyable way of getting back your pre-pregnancy figure. This is discussed further in Chapter 8.

The ball can also be used to just sit on. It may sound obvious but there are great benefits to replacing your office chair with a ball. In fact, physiotherapists have been arguing for years that we should replace chairs in offices and schools with balls. This is not only due to the benefits to our core strength and posture; studies have shown that sitting on a ball can improve concentration, especially in children. A 2003 study published in the American Journal of Occupational Therapy concluded that students with ADHD had improved behaviour and were able to focus and write more clearly when sitting on balls.

Whether you want to increase your fitness level, lose weight, tone muscles, increase flexibility or simply find a way to make exercising more enjoyable, there will be many exercise ball options available to you.

So, if you don't have a ball, it's time to go and get one and give it a name… as it will certainly become your new best friend!

BENEFITS AT A GLANCE

- O Affordable and easy to store.
- O Can be used as part of a fitness programme for toning, improving fitness levels, weight loss, increasing flexibility and posture.
- O An increased range of movement is possible due to the round shape of the ball.
- O Exercising on an unstable surface recruits deep stabilising muscles otherwise ignored.
- O Strengthens core muscles, which helps to prevent back and other common injuries.
- O Provides functional movement skills, enabling us to stay strong, flexible and independent into later life.
- O Adds interest to other workout forms such as yoga and Pilates.
- O Can be used to aid pregnancy and birthing.
- O Can be used as a chair, with the added benefit of improving posture and concentration.

CHAPTER ONE

GETTING STARTED

WHICH BALL?

With an extensive array of exercise balls on the market in different colours, sizes, durability and all with different names, it can be a little confusing when deciding which to buy.

The first thing to think about is size, as it is very important to buy the right ball for your height. Use the chart below as a general guide, although each ball company may specify something slightly different and ball sizes can vary, so always check the manufacturer's recommendations. If possible it is also a good idea to test the ball for size before buying. You can do this by sitting on the ball like a chair. When seated, your hips should be either level with your knees or just slightly higher. If you feel you are on the cusp between two sizes it is always better to go for the bigger ball and then just inflate it a little less.

Ball size guide

Your height	Ball size
Under 1.5m (4'11")	45 cm
1.5–1.6m (4'11"–5'4")	55 cm
1.65–1.8m (5'5"–5'10")	65 cm
Over 1.8m (5'11")	75 cm

Next make sure that the ball you are going to buy is made with burst-resistant material. This means that if for any reason you puncture your ball, instead of popping like a balloon, it will deflate slowly allowing you time to dismount safely. Try to avoid brands made from cheaper material that don't have this benefit.

Examine the balls on offer to you and try to choose one that looks sturdy and has a surface that looks like it will have a bit of grip.

INFLATING YOUR BALL

You may find that your ball comes packaged with a pump for inflation. If not, you can buy one specifically designed for the ball very cheaply online. Alternatively, as long as you have the correct adapters, you can use either an electric pump that plugs into a car lighter socket or an ordinary foot pump.

Ideally you want your ball to be quite firm, although if you are a beginner it is sometimes a good idea to start with the ball a little less inflated, as it offers more support and stability when softer. The firmer the ball, the more of a balance challenge the exercises will be. A good way to test that you have inflated your ball to the correct diameter, is to open a door by the correct number of centimetres and see if your ball fits into the gap.

When inflating your ball for the first time, some manufacturers recommend inflating to 70 per cent and leaving over night before fully inflating the next day. You will also find that your ball 'gives' a little after the first few days of use, so you may need to put a little more air in at this point.

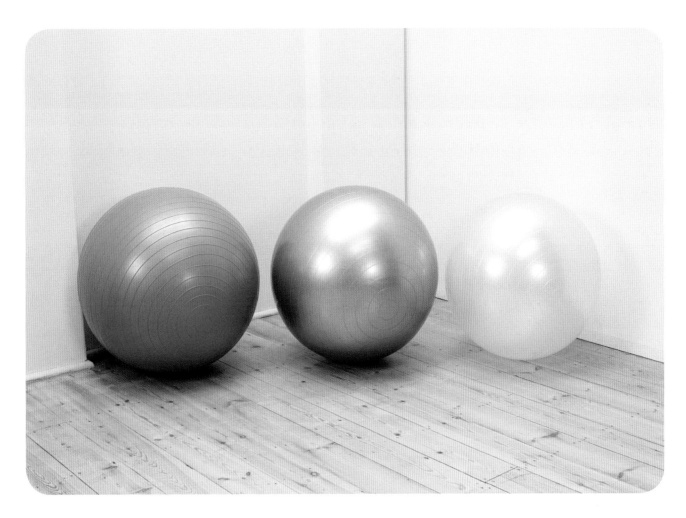

CARING FOR YOUR BALL

Before you start exercising with the ball, make sure the space around you is clean and free from any sharp objects or pieces of furniture that could damage it.

The ball is an extremely low maintenance piece of equipment and only needs a quick wipe down with soapy water every now and then.

HOW MUCH SPACE WILL I NEED?

How much space you need will depend entirely on what you intend to do with the ball. In an ideal world find a room to use where you have a body's length around your ball in all directions. This will enable you to do most exercises without constant re-adjustment of the ball. It is, however, possible to work in a smaller space, but this will require re-positioning the ball before you begin each exercise.

If you intend to try some of the aerobic moves and routines in the book (which I can highly recommend), you may need to be more aware of the things around you, such as any breakables, light fittings, etc. before you start throwing and bouncing the ball!

WILL I NEED OTHER EQUIPMENT OR SPECIAL CLOTHING?

You won't need to go out and buy special clothing for use with the ball, just make sure that you are wearing something loose and comfortable, but avoid anything that might get caught around the ball when you are moving. It is also a good idea to wear trousers that can roll up to your knees if necessary, as for some exercises you will need to be able to get a good grip on the ball with your legs. For most sections in the book I would advise working on the ball in bare feet, as trainers tend to get in the way. However, when working through the aerobics section, put your trainers back on, as they will help to absorb any impact from the floor, protecting you from injury.

One piece of equipment you will see me using throughout the book is a mat. This is primarily to make yourself more comfortable when lying or kneeling on the floor; it also provides a non-slip surface for you to work on. Although a mat is not a necessity, I would recommend that you get one. A yoga-type mat is perfect; make sure it is the non-slip variety. If your budget doesn't extend to a mat right now, then don't worry, you can improvise by using a rug or carpeted area you already have in your home.

You will also notice that Chapter 2 has a section dedicated to using weights with the ball. If you have some hand weights, then great – you will need anything from a 1–4lb weight depending on the exercise. If you don't happen to have any weights stashed in the back of the closet that's fine too. At the beginning of that section I will explain how to make a perfectly good set of your own.

There has been lots of other paraphernalia designed to be used with the ball, such as stands, carry straps, resistance bands, chair frames etc. Some of these are of course useful but none are essential.

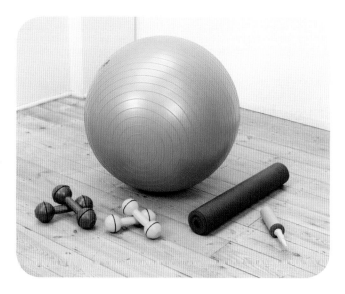

BEFORE YOU START CHECKLIST

O If you have any concerns about your health, if you are pregnant or if you are receiving medical treatment or medication of any kind, it is always best to consult your doctor before starting any exercise programme.

O Ensure that you are wearing comfortable clothing that is not restrictive to your movement.

O Ensure that the space around you is clear from any objects that may damage your ball and that you have ideally one body's length of space around you in all directions.

O Ensure you are working on a comfortable non-slip surface – preferably a mat.

O Ensure you have had a few minutes to acclimatise yourself to moving on the ball before moving on to the set exercises.

BALL ACCLIMATISATION

If you have never had a go on a ball before now, I suggest that you spend a few minutes acclimatising your body to the ball. This will allow you to get a feel for how the ball moves when you change your weight and position and to gain a little confidence before beginning any specific movements.

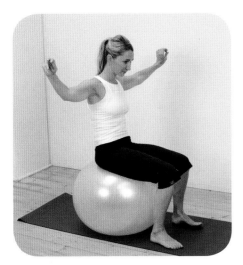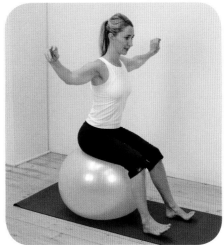

Start by sitting on the ball and have a play with it to see how it feels when you push it to the right and left, forwards and backwards. You will start to get a sense of your centre of gravity and how far off balance you can allow yourself to go without toppling off completely.

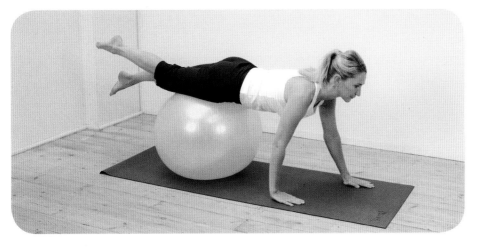

Now try lying over the ball on your hand and knees. Once again have a play with your weight, test how far you can walk out onto your hands, get a sense of your own balance limitations on the ball.

FINDING AND MAINTAINING NEUTRAL SPINE ALIGNMENT

When working on the ball, if we are to avoid injury and strengthen our deep core muscles, it is crucial that we work (where appropriate) in a neutral spine position. Maintaining neutral spine just means that we acknowledge the natural curves that are in our spine: curving in at the neck (cervical spine), curving out on the upper back (thoracic spine) and in again at the lower back (lumbar spine). These curves are there to act as shock absorbers for our body.

We mustn't allow these to become over-exaggerated when getting into certain positions, as this may put unnecessary pressure on the spine and could lead to injury. In the next exercises we are going to look at making sure our spine is in a neutral position when taking up different stances with and without the ball. We will also learn how to use the abdominal muscles to secure the spine so that we can move around on the ball without compromising that neutral position.

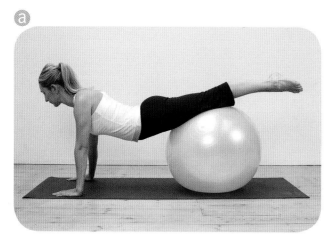

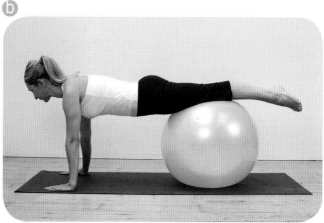

Example of incorrect posture. This shows an over-exaggerated curve of the lower back, putting strain on the spine

Correct posture. This shows neutral spine alignment.

We will start by finding our neutral spine position without the ball in a standing position, and then seated on the ball. The following exercises are worth doing in front of a full-length mirror if possible. This way you will be able to see the very subtle movements of the spine and be able to visually remember what your neutral position looks like.

STANDING NEUTRAL POSITION

1 **a** Stand with your feet hip width apart, knees slightly relaxed and your arms down by your sides.

2 Transfer your weight forwards onto your toes **b** and then back onto your heels. **c** Keep this motion going, gradually making the movement smaller and smaller. You should start to feel a central position where you feel most centred and on balance, stop here.

3 Make sure that your shoulders are relaxed in this position and that your neck is in line with the rest of your spine; your chin should neither be lifted nor dropped.

4 Now keeping your weight centred, start tilting your pelvis forwards **d** and back **e**, again gradually making the movement smaller and smaller until you begin to feel a place in the middle where your pelvis feels heavy and most centred, stop here. This is your standing neutral spine position.

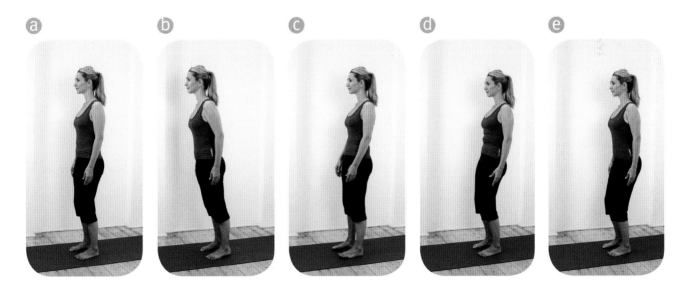

a b c d e

SEATED NEUTRAL POSITION

1 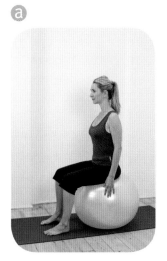 Start seated on your ball with your feet hip width apart. Make sure that you are sitting directly on your sitting bones (these are the bony bits underneath your bottom that you can feel when sitting on a hard floor).

2 Imagine lifting tall, lengthening through the crown of your head, shoulders pushing down.

3 Tilt your pelvis forwards 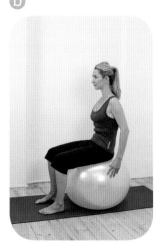 and then backwards 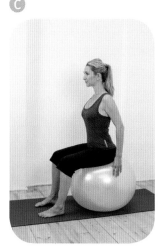, gradually making the movement smaller and smaller until you come to rest in the position where you feel your spine is most centred. This is your seated neutral position.

ⓐ

ⓑ

ⓒ

TIP

Because of our natural body shape you will find that when seated, the natural curve of the spine is less than when you are standing.

ENGAGING THE CORE

We now need to bring our 'core' muscles into play if we have any chance of maintaining our neutral spine position once some movement is thrown into the equation.

The core muscles refer not only to your stomach muscles but also to the transversus abdominus, multifidus, diaphragm and pelvic floor all of which are located around the abdominal and pelvic area. By using all of these muscles you gain maximum stability around the abdominal and lower back region, reducing strain.

The following exercises use visualisations by which you can learn how to 'engage' your core muscles. This is a very important step to try and master before beginning your work with the ball.

ENGAGING THE CORE: EXERCISE 1

1   Start in your standing neutral spine position, imagine that you are wearing a belt around your abdomen and it has ten holes in it. Take a deep breath in and, as you breathe out, imagine you are doing up the belt to the tenth notch, so it is as tight as it can go. Now loosen the belt to the third notch and keep it here. This is now a 30 per cent contraction, which is about right for you to be able to move freely but still have enough abdominal and spine stabilisation.

ENGAGING THE CORE: EXERCISE 2

1   This time you are going to learn to draw up the pelvic floor muscles. To get a sense of what these muscles feel like, imagine you are passing urine and you want to stop mid-flow. Practise this a few times so you can really feel the pelvic floor muscles working.

2   Now you know where these muscles are, imagine that you have an elevator with ten floors that runs from your pelvis to the bottom of your rib cage. Now take a deep breath in and as you breathe out draw the elevator all the way up to the tenth floor. Now allow the elevator to come back down to the third floor and keep it here. This again is your 30 per cent contraction that you are aiming to maintain.

You can use either of these visualisations each time you are asked to 'engage your core' or, when you have had a bit more practice, you can try using them both at the same time. Although it might feel very unnatural if it is not something you are used to, it should soon become second nature and you will even find yourself automatically engaging when sitting or standing in your everyday life.

BASE POSITIONS

The following positions are used over and over again with the ball. These are called the base positions and you will notice as you work through the book that most exercises either start or pass through one of these positions. If you are new to the ball, I would thoroughly recommend that you have a go at each of these positions and master getting in and out of them before moving on to the exercises.

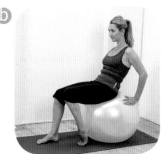
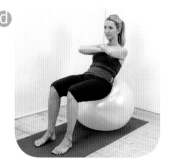

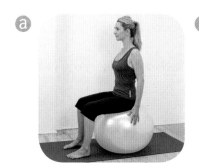
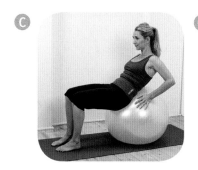

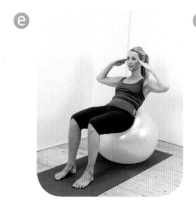
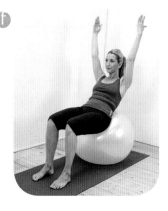

1. SEATED BASE POSITION

1　**a** Sit on the ball with your feet hip width apart, your knees over your ankle joints and your arms resting by your sides. Make sure that your spine is in the neutral position.

2. SEATED WALKING

This is a transitional movement that we use to get in and out of other positions.

1　**b** From your seated base position, start walking your feet forward allowing the ball to start rolling up your spine. **c** Stop when the ball is resting in your lower back.

3　Now walk your feet back in, allowing your body to roll back up into the seated base position.

3. INCLINE POSITION

1　From your seated base position, use seated walking to walk out until the ball is once again resting in your lower back. Make sure your feet are flat on the floor and hip width apart and that your neck is in a neutral position.

2　There are three different arm positions you can use here; across your chest **d**, hands to temples **e** or arms extended overhead **f**.

4. SUPINE POSITION WITH BACK OR NECK SUPPORT

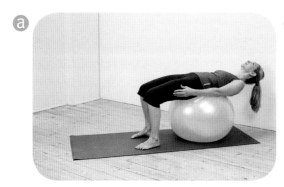

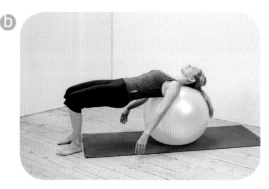

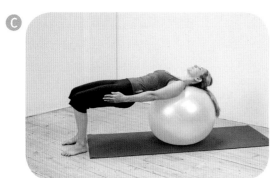

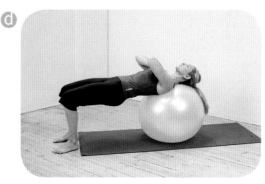

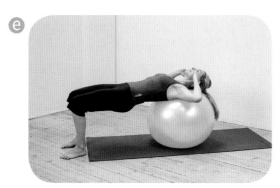

1 **a** From your incline position on the ball, take your weight a little further back on the ball by walking your feet in a few steps, so the ball is resting in your lower back. This is supine with back support.

2 **b** Now walk your feet forwards, allowing the ball to roll up the spine until it is resting underneath the back of your neck. Keep your hips lifted in this position so that your torso is parallel to the floor. This is your supine position with neck support; sometimes this is also referred to as the suspended bridge position.

3 In both supine positions you can either place your arms by your sides **c**, across your chest **d** or on your temples **e**.

5. SIDE LYING POSITION

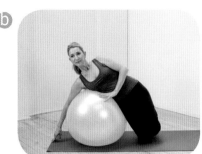

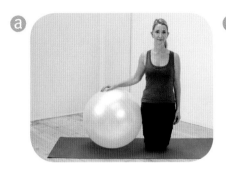

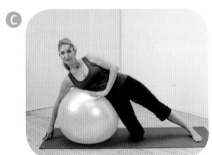

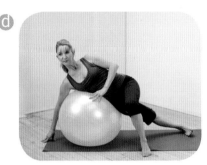

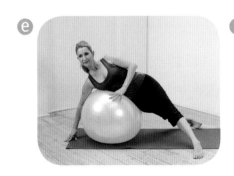

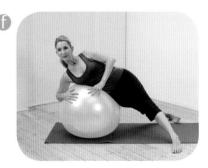

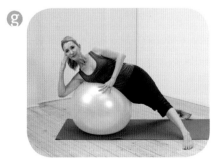

1 ⓐ Start kneeling on the floor with the ball by your right side.

2 ⓑ Lengthen your body sideways over the ball, making sure that you keep your hips square on to the front, reaching your right arm over the ball towards the floor.

3 ⓒ For the most basic leg position you can use here, extend your top leg out to the side, keeping the underneath leg bent.

4 ⓓ For the second leg position, bend your top leg, placing the foot flat on the floor in front of the line of the body, then extend your underneath leg.

5 ⓔ For the scissor position (which is the most difficult), extend both legs so that your top leg is scissored over the bottom one, the weight evenly distributed between your two feet.

6 To make this position even more challenging you can place your underneath hand either on the ball ⓕ or on your temple. ⓖ

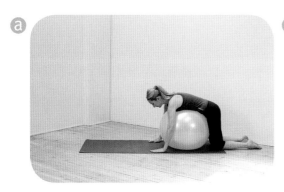

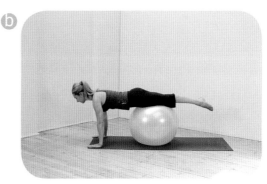

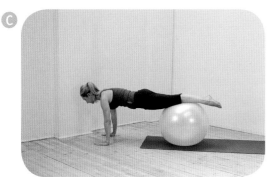

1 ⓐ There are three variations to this position. For trunk support, start kneeling on the floor facing your ball, place your hands on the floor over the ball so you are in an all fours position.

2 ⓑ For hip support, walk yourself out with your hands a little further over the ball, allowing the ball to roll down your body. This is called prone walking. Stop when the ball is resting underneath your hips.

3 ⓒ For lower leg support, keep walking further out on the ball until it is resting underneath your lower leg. The further you walk out, the more difficult the position will become. Only walk out on the ball as far as you are able to ensure your spine is in a neutral position and you don't start sagging in the middle.

CORRECT BREATHING

Breathing is something that most of us give little thought to, even though it is essential to life. Our body is wired to automatically take in oxygen which then gets transported around the body by our blood cells. During exercise this is how we oxygenate our hard-working muscles and supply them with nutrient rich blood. When we exhale, we get rid of toxins and gases such as carbon dioxide that our body doesn't need.

Breathing correctly is essential, therefore, if you are to sustain high intensity exercise for any extended period of time. If we don't manage our breathing properly, the muscles will not receive the essential oxygen they need to keep working at a higher intensity level. Generally speaking you will naturally fall into breathing out on the exertion phase of an exercise and should try and find a natural rhythm of coordinating your breath with movement. It is important to avoid taking shallow breaths, which only work half your total lung capacity, when you start to get tired.

When taking part in aerobic exercise (by aerobic I mean exercise that makes your rate of respiration increase and makes you hot and sweaty), your rate of breath can be a good way of measuring your intensity level. Instead of using a heart rate monitor or taking your pulse, the American Heart Association recommends using a conversational pace as an alternative to gauge exercise intensity:

1. If you can talk easily when exercising you are not working hard enough.
2. If you get out of breath quickly and have to stop to catch your breath you need to ease off a little.

When we are working on the ball and placing our body in positions where we need to maintain our neutral spine, our breathing has to be slightly more thought out. In order to offer the greatest support to the lower back and pelvis we of course need to 'engage the core', therefore it is difficult to breathe deep into the abdomen whilst maintaining our 30 per cent contraction. We need to learn a new breathing technique where we direct the breath into the ribcage.

BREATHING PREPARATIONS

These exercises will teach you how to direct the breath into different areas of the ribcage in order to maintain neutral spine position and core contraction.

BREATHING EXERCISE 1

Direct the breath to the back of the ribcage while maintaining your core contraction.

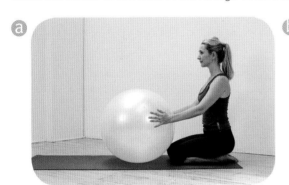 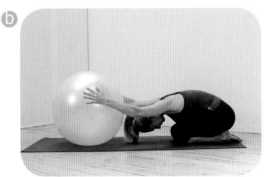

1 ⓐ Start kneeling in front of your ball with your hands placed on the outside of your ball.

2 ⓑ Now roll your ball forwards, extending your arms in front of you. Round your back and rest your head forwards in a relaxed position. Engage your core to 30 per cent.

3 Inhale through your nose, sending your breath into the back of your ribcage, then exhale through your mouth.

4 Stay here for a while taking slow controlled breaths; really feel the back of the ribcage expand each time it is filled with air.

TIP

Imagine you are a fish breathing through its gills. Make sure you fully inhale and exhale the breath and are not creating tension elsewhere in the body.

BREATHING EXERCISE 2

Direct the breath to the back of the ribcage while maintaining neutral spine and your core contraction.

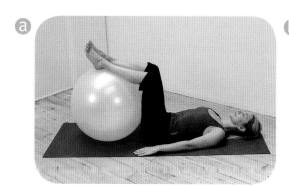 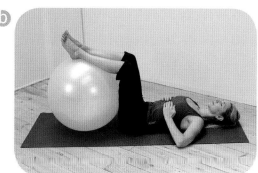

1 **a** Start lying on the floor with your legs placed on the ball. Make sure your knees are directly over your hips and are hip width apart. Your spine should be in a neutral position here, so you should have a slight curve in the lower back – just enough to slide a piece of paper under, nothing more. Engage your core contraction by thinking of pulling in your belt to the third notch and drawing up the lift to the third floor to maintain this position in the spine and pelvis.

2 **b** Place your hands onto your ribcage with your fingers pointing inwards. Think about settling into a natural breathing pace, directing the breath into the back of the ribcage. When you inhale, your fingers should part as the ribcage expands, and when you exhale, they should come back together. Continue for a couple of minutes.

TIP

When you inhale think about the drawing up of the pelvic floor muscles, or your lift visualisation. When you exhale think about re-establishing the abdominal to spine connection, the doing up of the belt.

BREATHING EXERCISE 3

Directing the breath into the side of the ribcage while side-lying on the ball and maintaining your core contraction. This exercise also opens up and stretches each lung in turn.

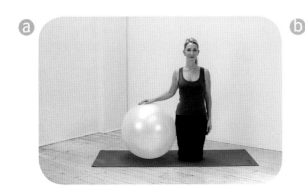
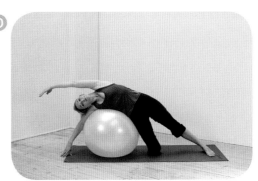

1 **ⓐ** Start by kneeling with the ball on your right side. Engage your core contraction.

2 **ⓑ** Now reach your right arm over the ball, allowing your body to relax onto the ball. Extend your left arm over your head and your left leg out to the side.

3 Breathe in through your nose, directing the breath into the left side of your ribcage, and then breathe out through your mouth. Take 5–6 breaths in this position, then repeat on the other side.

TIP

Make sure that your body stays in alignment as it is draped over the ball. Your hips and shoulders should be square on to the front.

WARMING UP

Why should I warm up? I have heard this question asked so many times over the years. The warm up is probably the most underrated part of any exercise programme and therefore the part that is most likely to get axed when time is short. I cannot stress enough, however, the benefits of a proper warm up appropriate to the exercise you are about to take part in.

Warming up is designed to prepare the body for the demands of the exercise that is to follow. The idea is to increase circulation throughout the body and your overall body temperature in a gradual manner. As your circulatory system starts to pump oxygen-rich blood to your working muscles they begin to become more pliable. You could think of your muscles as a piece of play dough – when it's cold it tends to break away quite easily when pulled, and yet with a bit of gentle warming up it becomes quite pliable and stretchy. Cold muscles are not supple, do not absorb shock or impact well and are therefore very susceptible to injury.

The gradual increase of activity also helps to prepare the heart, avoiding a rapid increase in blood pressure. It primes your nerve-to-muscle pathways to be ready for exercise and synovial fluid is released to lubricate the joints and again make muscles more supple and elastic. Your body will even go through some hormonal changes during the warm up, increasing production of the hormones responsible for regulation of energy production, making more carbohydrates and fatty acids available for increased energy.

Perhaps the most overlooked reason of all to embark on a warm up is to mentally prepare. It helps to clear the mind of everyday thoughts and dilemmas and allows you to focus on the job at hand. I can honestly say that on the occasions that I have failed to have a proper warm up I have found it incredibly hard to focus my mind away from everyday chores and my motivation is certainly nowhere to be found!

As you make your way through this book you and your ball will be taking part in many different styles of exercise. For each of these the requirements of the warm up are slightly different. All have a common link, which is to prepare the body for what is to come, so you will need to adapt your warm-up exercises accordingly. The important elements of a warm up are to increase your body temperature so that you feel warm, to mobilise the joints and to have a 'prep stretch' for the muscles. This means a gentle stretch just as preparation, but you shouldn't be forcing a deep stretch or trying to increase flexibility.

You can choose whether you would like to simply work through some or all of the exercises listed here, or if you would rather follow the routine I have put together for you at the end of the chapter. Whatever you choose, try to make sure that your warm up lasts between 5–10 minutes. Some of the exercise forms in the book do not require a separate warm up. In the yoga section (Chapter 5) and the Pilates section (Chapter 4) your warm up will be about focusing the mind and breath and will be explained within each chapter. In Chapter 8 (Pregnancy, Birthing and Beyond), we will examine how to adapt the exercises depending on your stage.

WARM-UP EXERCISES

LOOK RIGHT AND LEFT

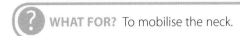 **WHAT FOR?** To mobilise the neck.

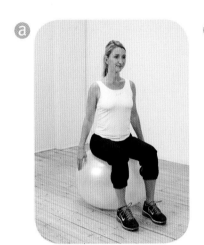

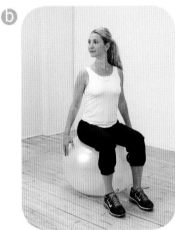

1 **a** Start seated on your ball in neutral spine position with your feet hip width apart on the floor, your knees directly over ankles and your arms relaxed down by your sides.

2 **b** Keeping your nose level, turn your head slowly so that you are looking over your right shoulder.

3 Now turn your head back to the centre.

4 Repeat on the left.

INCREASE THE LEVEL

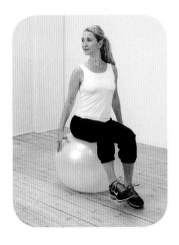

To add a balance challenge to this exercise, try it again with your right leg lifted a few inches off the floor. Once you have looked in both directions, swap legs.

TIPS

- Try to ensure that there is no movement anywhere else in the body as the head looks from side to side. This is a really good opportunity to feel your core contraction fixing your torso in place.
- Imagine your nose is a piece of chalk and you are drawing a steady line in a semi-circle around your head.

WHAT FOR? To mobilise the pelvis.

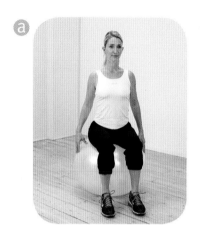

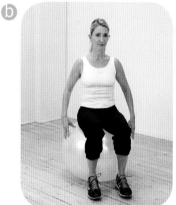

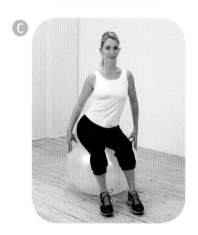

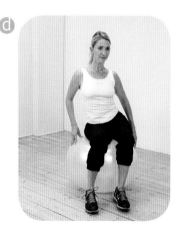

1 Start seated on your ball in your neutral spine position with your feet hip width apart on the floor, your knees directly over ankles and your arms relaxed down by your sides.

2 Now push your hips forwards then continue in a circle around to the right, then to the back, finally to the left side until you have completed a full circle and have returned to your neutral position.

3 Repeat, taking your circle to the left side first.

INCREASE THE LEVEL

1 Start in your neutral position as before.
2 This time, starting to the right, draw a 'figure of 8' with your hips.

TIPS

- Try to keep your knees and ankles stabilised throughout the exercise.
- Keep your core contraction in place; this will ensure you do not overarch the spine.
- If necessary lightly touch the sides of your ball for increased stability.

SEATED ARM CIRCLES

? **WHAT FOR?** To mobilise the shoulder joints and to challenge your neutral spine position.

 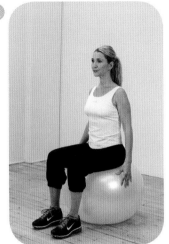

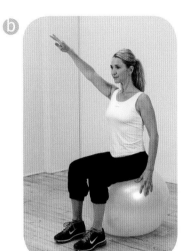

1 Start seated on the centre of your ball in neutral spine position with your feet hip width apart, knees directly over ankles and arms by your sides.

2 **b** Circle your right arm backwards until it comes full circle back to your ball.

3 Repeat, this time circling your left arm backwards.

4 Now start with your right arm again, this time circling forwards. Repeat on the left.

INCREASE THE LEVEL

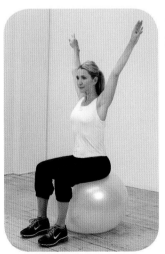

1 Start in neutral as before.
2 This time circle both arms together, first backwards and then forwards.

TIPS

- Use your lift and belt visualisations as discussed earlier in the chapter to stabilise your torso while the arms are moving. This is especially challenging when moving both arms together.
- Try to avoid any twisting of the spine – your hips and shoulders should stay square on to the front.

WHAT FOR? To open up the ribcage and mobilise the torso.

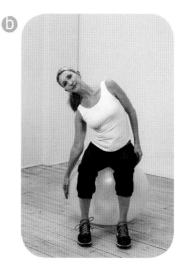

1 Start seated on your ball in neutral spine position with your feet hip width apart, knees directly over ankles and arms by your sides.

2 Keeping your shoulders square on to the front, reach your right hand down the ball as far as is comfortable , then return to your neutral position.

3 Repeat on the left.

 INCREASE THE LEVEL

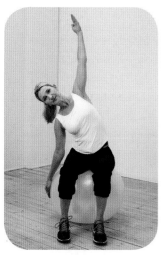

1 Start in neutral as before.
2 As you reach your right hand down the ball, simultaneously reach your left arm up above your head.
3 Return to your neutral position, then repeat on the other side.

TIPS

- Try to keep your head in line with the rest of your spine as you bend to the side. This will avoid any strain in the neck.
- Only reach as far to the side as is comfortable and which allows you to maintain your core contraction.

BOUNCING ON THE BALL

? WHAT FOR? To increase body temperature, heart rate and mobilise the knee and hip joints.

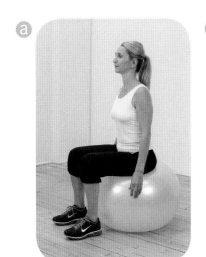
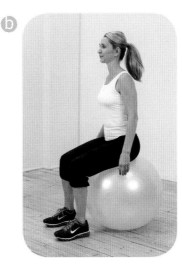

1 **a** Start seated on the centre of your ball in neutral spine position with your feet hip width apart, knees directly over ankles and arms by your sides.

2 **b** Start bouncing up and down by pushing your feet into the floor, allowing the bottom to come slightly off the ball, but not so far that your ball will roll from under you.

3 Keep breathing and stay relaxed as you bounce.

INCREASE THE LEVEL

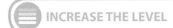

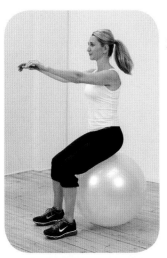

1 Start bouncing as before.
2 Swing your arms in front of you to eye level, then behind your back as you continue to bounce.

TIPS

- Keep your knees directly over ankles when bouncing.
- Make sure you do not bend or twist the spine as you bounce.
- Bounce gently at first, and then increase in vigour as you grow more confident with the ball.

? WHAT FOR? To test your balance and mobilise the knee joints.

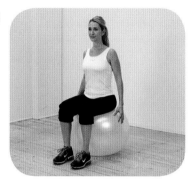 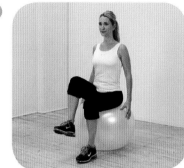 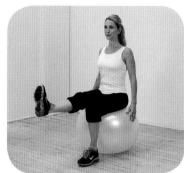

1 **a** Start seated on your ball in neutral spine position with your feet hip width apart, knees directly over ankles and hands lightly touching the sides of the ball.

2 **b** Lift your right foot a few inches off the floor.

3 **c** Now extend the right leg in front of you, whilst maintaining your balance.

4 Bend the knee again as in **b**, and lower the foot back to the floor.

5 Repeat on the left.

INCREASE THE LEVEL

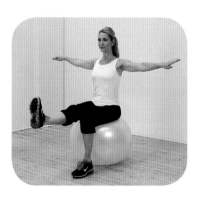

1 Start in your neutral position as before, but this time take your arms out to the sides.

2 Repeat the exercise alternating legs as before, maintaining the position of the arms.

TIPS

- Imagine that you have a piece of string extending from the crown of your head and someone is pulling you up towards the ceiling making you as tall as possible. Maintain this visualisation as you lift each leg off the floor.
- Start by keeping your leg low, you can increase the height once you gain confidence and balance.

HALF JACKS

? WHAT FOR? To increase body temperature, heart rate and mobilise the hip and shoulder joints.

 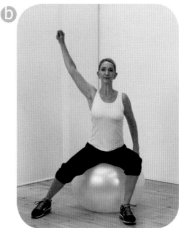

1 **a** Start seated on the ball in neutral spine position, feet hip width apart, knees over hips, arms down by your sides.

2 Start a bouncing motion, on the first bounce extend your right arm and right leg sideways, **b** on the second bounce bring them back to the starting position.

3 Repeat on the left, keeping the bounces in a steady rhythm.

≡ INCREASE THE LEVEL

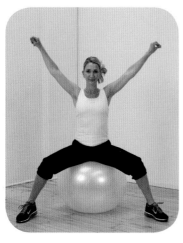

1 From your seated position, on your first bounce jump both your legs out to the side at the same time as extending your arms out to the side.

2 On the second bounce, jump the legs back to the starting position and bring your arms back to your sides, ready to go again.

TIPS

- Make sure as you move your legs out to the side, the knees stay facing the same direction as your toes.
- Bounce gently at first building up vigour as you grow in confidence.
- Keep your spine in neutral, avoid bending or twisting as you bounce.

? **WHAT FOR?** To increase body temperature, heart rate and mobilise the knee joints.

 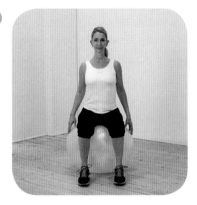 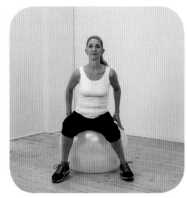 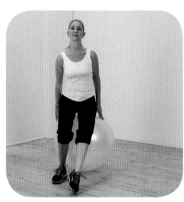

1 **a** Start seated on the ball in neutral spine position. Check your feet are hip width apart, knees over ankles, and arms down by your sides with your hands lightly supported on the ball.

2 Step your right foot to the side taking the weight onto it, **b** and then tap your left foot in front of you. **c**

3 Repeat on the other side, using a bouncing action as you change from side to side.

INCREASE THE LEVEL

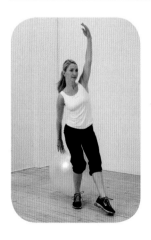

1 Start in your seated neutral spine position as before and start by stepping the right foot to the side and taking the weight onto it.

2 This time as you tap the left foot in front of you, reach your left arm forwards, take some of your weight into your right hand so it is pushing into the ball and allow your bottom to come slightly off the ball.

3 Repeat on the other side, again trying to initiate a bouncing motion.

TIPS

- Keep the spine in its neutral position and your core contraction activated as you move from side to side.
- Bounce gently at first, building up vigour as you grow in confidence.
- Use the hand-to-ball contact to help stabilise you as you move from side to side.

? **WHAT FOR?** To increase body temperature, heart rate and mobilise the hip and knee joints.

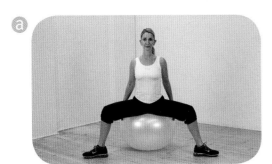

1 **a** Start seated on your ball in neutral spine position. Place your feet in a wide position, knees bent, turning your legs out so that your feet and knees are pointing out in a 45-degree angle (or as far as you feel comfortable). Take your weight forwards onto the front of the ball, stretching into the hips.

2 **b** Roll your weight over to the right side, bending the right knee further making sure that the knee stays over the line of the foot, and extending the left leg.

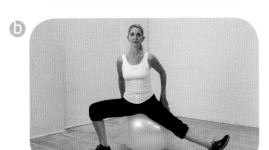

3 Now push yourself all the way over to the other side. You should now have your left knee bent and your right leg straight.

4 Continue to push from side to side allowing the ball to roll underneath you.

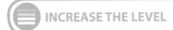
INCREASE THE LEVEL

1 Start your rocks from side to side as before.
2 As your right leg bends, move your arms across your body so they are pointing towards your left outstretched leg.
3 As you change sides, bending your left leg, move your arms across the body to point towards your right extended leg.
4 Keep changing from side to side in a steady rhythm.

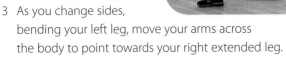

TIPS

- Always keep your knees pointing over the line of the feet and don't allow your knee to come further forwards than your ankle joint.
- By keeping your weight at the front of the ball as you move from side to side, your legs will do more work and therefore see more benefit.
- Make sure you stay facing square on to the front if you introduce the arm movement. This avoids any unnecessary twisting of the spine.

WHAT FOR? To increase body temperature, heart rate and mobilise the hip and knee joints.

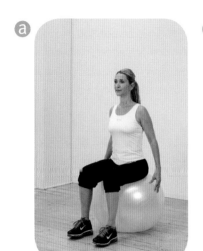

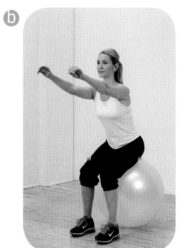

1 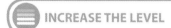 Start seated on your ball in neutral spine position with the feet hip width apart, knees directly over ankles, arms by your sides.

2 Push your feet into the floor, activating your thigh muscles as if you are going to stand up, but instead come up until your bottom just lifts an inch from the ball, then sit back down. As you lift up, raise your arms to eye level ⓑ, and relax them down again as you lower.

INCREASE THE LEVEL

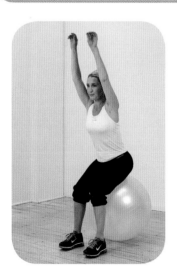

Perform the exercise as before, but this time raise your arms up above your head.

TIPS

- Don't lift too far off the ball to ensure it doesn't roll out from underneath you.
- Make sure your knees stay over the line of your ankles to avoid pressure on the knee joints.
- Keep your core contraction activated to protect the lower back.

WHAT FOR? To increase body temperature, heart rate and mobilise the hip and knee joints.

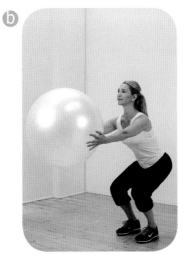

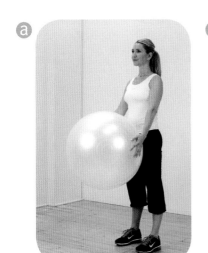

1 (a) Start standing in neutral position with your ball held in both hands, activating your core contraction. Ensure your feet are hip width apart and knees slightly soft.

2 (b) Bend your knees and sit yourself back, as if you intend to sit into a chair. Simultaneously lift the ball forwards to chest height.

3 Straighten your knees, bringing yourself back to your starting position and at the same time lower the ball back down.

4 Repeat at a rhythmical pace.

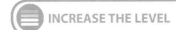 INCREASE THE LEVEL

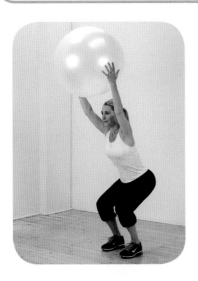

Start as before, this time raising your arms up until they are level with your forehead.

TIPS

- Ensure your knees do not bend lower than a 90-degree angle.
- As you bend, keep your knees directly over your ankles and make sure they stay hip width apart.
- Keep your abdominals activated as you squat, making sure that you do not arch the lower back.

'FIGURE OF 8' ARM CIRCLES

WHAT FOR? To increase body temperature, heart rate and mobilise the shoulder joints.

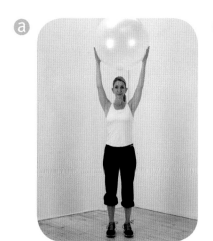 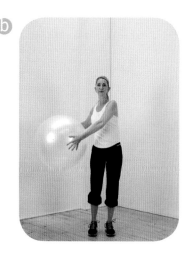 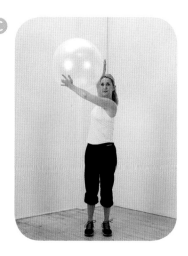

1 **a** Start standing in neutral position with your ball held in both hands above your head. Activate your core contraction. Ensure your feet are hip width apart and knees slightly soft.

2 Swing your arms down so the ball passes your right hip, **b** continuing the circle all the way around until your arms are back above your head, **c** immediately swing down again this time with the ball passing your left hip before returning to above your head completing the 'figure of 8' movement.

INCREASE THE LEVEL

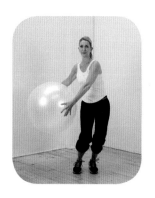

Complete the movement as before, this time as your arms swing downwards, bend your knees and as your arms come back overhead, straighten them.

TIPS

- Ensure you maintain your core contraction throughout the sequence to stabilise the position of the torso.
- Try releasing your breath as your arms swing down and inhaling as they return above your head.
- Start the exercise slowly and try to increase speed as you master the 'figure of 8' movement.

SEATED HAMSTRING STRETCH

? **WHAT FOR?** To stretch the hamstring muscles in the back of the legs, preparing them for the exercises to come.

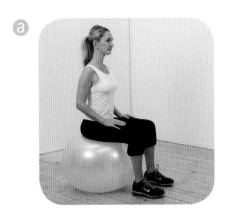 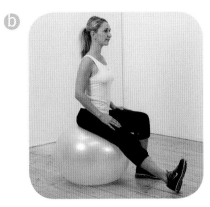 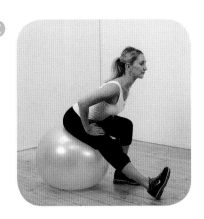

1 **a** Start seated on the ball in your neutral position with the feet hip width apart, knees directly over ankles, hands placed lightly on your thighs.

2 **b** Extend your right leg, placing your heel on the floor in front of you.

3 Now tilt your body forwards as far as is comfortable until you feel a stretch up the back of your right leg. **c** Hold the stretch for up to 30 seconds then repeat on the left.

INCREASE THE LEVEL

Repeat the exercise as before. This time as you tilt the torso forwards, take hold of your right toe with your right hand and gently pull the foot towards you. This will increase the intensity of the stretch.

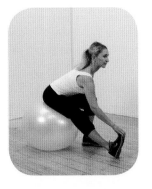

TIPS

- Try to think about relaxing into the stretch rather than forcing it.
- Only stretch as far as is comfortable, at this point the stretch is for warming up purposes and is not intended to be too deep.

STANDING FOOT TAPS WITH CHEST PRESS ARMS

? WHAT FOR? To increase the body temperature, heart rate and mobilise the shoulders, knees and hips.

1 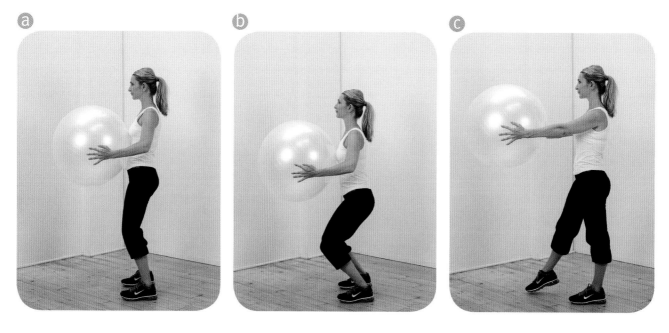 **a** Start standing with your feet wider than hip width apart and your ball held in both hands in front of your chest. Ensure your knees are soft and your core contraction is activated.

2 Bend both of your knees **b** then extend them taking your weight onto your left leg and tapping your right foot to the side. At the same time push the ball forwards, straightening your arms at chest height. **c**

3 Bend both knees again and bring the ball back in to your chest **d** and extend the knees again, this time taking your weight onto your right leg and tapping the left foot to the side. **e**

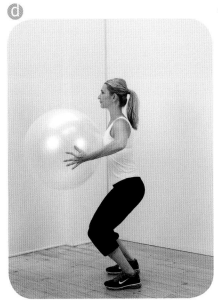

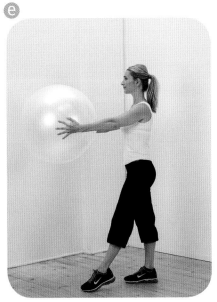

TIPS

- Make sure your knees are staying aligned above your ankles when bending the knees.
- When your arms are extended make sure you don't lock the elbows, instead keep a softness in the joint.
- Try to coordinate your breathing so that you exhale as you straighten the legs and arms.

INCREASE THE LEVEL

Repeat the exercise as before, but this time when you extend your arms, push them up above your head rather than forwards.

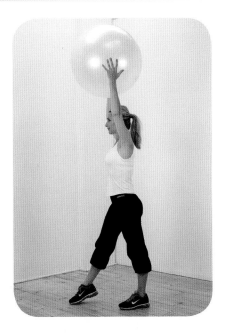

WHAT FOR? To stretch the deltoid muscles of the shoulder.

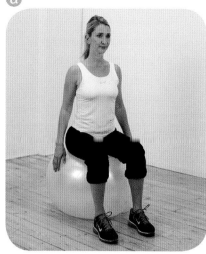

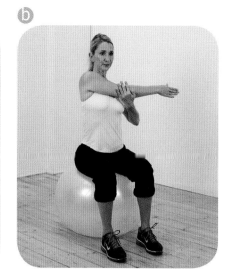

TIPS

- Only take the stretch as far as is comfortable.
- Ensure your body stays facing forwards to avoid any twisting in the spine.

1 ⓐ Start seated on the ball with your feet hip width apart, knees over ankles, your spine in neutral position. Activate your core contraction.

2 ⓑ Reach your right arm across your body, place your left hand on your right elbow and use your hand to pull the arm in towards your chest.

3 Hold the stretch for up to 30 seconds, then release the arm and repeat on the other side.

TRICEP STRETCH

 WHAT FOR? To stretch the tricep muscles in the back of the arms.

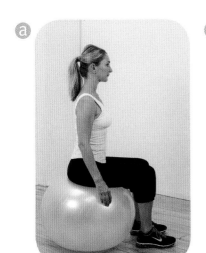

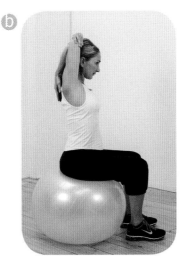

1 **a** Start seated on the ball with your feet hip width apart, knees over ankles, and your spine in neutral position. Activate your core contraction.

2 **b** Reach your right hand down your back as far as you can and gently push back on the elbow with your left hand.

3 Hold the stretch for up to 30 seconds. Release the arm and repeat on the other side.

INCREASE THE LEVEL

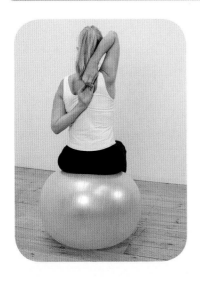

If you are flexible in the shoulders, instead of pushing back on the elbow, you can try to reach the other hand up the back and link the fingers together.

TIPS

- Try not to allow your back to arch as you reach down the back.
- Only push back on the arm as far as is comfortable.

? **WHAT FOR?** To stretch the quadricep muscles in the front of the thigh.

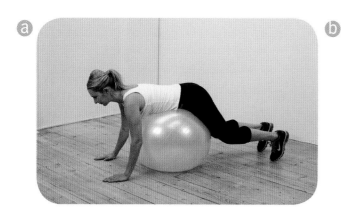

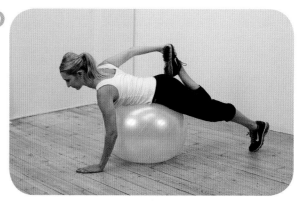

1 **a** Start on your hands and knees over the ball. Walk out slightly, taking the knees off the floor so that the weight is even between your hands and feet.

2 **b** Bring your right heel towards your bottom and take hold of the foot with your right hand. Keep both hips in contact with the ball.

3 Push your hips into the ball to increase the stretch. Hold for up to 30 seconds.

4 Relax the leg back down. Repeat on the left.

TIPS

- Try not to strain the upper body to reach the foot. If you struggle, use a towel or dressing gown belt wrapped around the foot to help you to reach.
- Keep the hips and shoulders square to the floor.
- Focus down to the floor to keep the neck in line with the rest of the spine.

WHAT FOR? To stretch the hip flexors, the glutes (your bottom) and your hamstrings.

 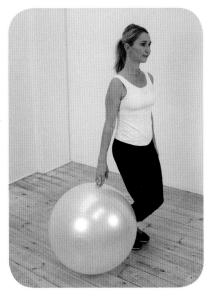

 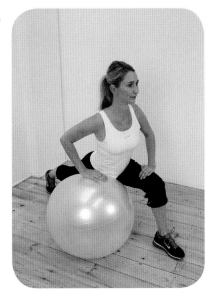

TIPS

- Make sure that your front knee stays directly over your ankle when your leg is in the lunge position. This will avoid putting excessive pressure on the knee joint.
- Once in position, push the hip of the extended leg into the ball to feel the stretch increase into the hip flexor.

1 Start standing with the ball placed on the floor next to your right foot.

2 Slide your right leg backwards into a lunge position. At the same time use your right hand to place the ball underneath your right hip.

3 Hold the stretch for up to 30 seconds, using the ball to offer as much or little support as you need.

4 Come back up to a standing position, repeat on the left.

WARM-UP ROUTINE

I have put together a fun routine from a selection of the above exercises. Of course you could have lots of fun choreographing your own warm-up routine, either from the exercises listed above or by adding some of your own. Find some upbeat music that is to your liking, pop it on and here we go!

Look right and left (page 29)
x16 in time with the music

Seated arm circles (page 31)
Circle right and then left

Hip circles (page 30)
1 slowly each side, 4 fast each side

Bouncing on the ball (page 33)
x16 Bounce in time with the music for 16 counts

Seated side reaches (page 32)
Reach right and then left

Seated one-leg extensions (page 34)
x4 Extend right and left

Seated arm circles (page 31)
Circle right and then left

Bouncing on the ball (page 33)
x16 Bounce in time with the music for 16 counts

Seated side reaches (page 32)
Reach right and left

Seated hamstring stretch (page 41)
Stretch each leg, holding for 15–30 seconds

Half jacks (page 35)

Repeat 8 times on the right, 8 on the left then 16 alternating legs

Shoulder stretch (page 44)

Stretch each shoulder, holding for 10–15 seconds

Tricep stretch (page 45)

Stretch each arm, holding for 10–15 seconds

Rocks from side to side (page 37)

×16 alternating sides

Foot taps (page 36)

×16 alternating legs

Half stand ups (page 38)

×16 staying standing on the last one

'Figure of 8' arm circles (page 40)

×8 alternating sides

Squats (page 39)

×16

Standing foot taps with chest press arms (page 42)

×16 alternating legs

Quad stretch (page 46)

Stretch each leg, holding up to 30 seconds

Lunge with ball support (page 47)

Lunge each side, holding for up to 30 seconds

'Figure of 8' arm circles (page 40)

×8 alternating sides

Squats (page 39)

×16

Standing foot taps with chest press arms (page 42)

×16 alternating legs

CHAPTER TWO

TONING AND STRENGTHENING WITH THE BALL

INTRODUCTION

This chapter is all about firming up the wobbly bits, strengthening the weak bits and improving your overall body image and functionality. The versatility of the ball means it can be used as a weight, a bench or a surface to enable positions otherwise unattainable or usually only possible with a partner.

Throughout the chapter we are going to look at exercises specific to each body part, allowing you to choose which areas you would like to work on. Remember, though, that the body is a whole integrated unit and needs balance. If you only work the muscles in your back, your opposing muscles in the chest will eventually become weak, so try to create a plan where throughout the course of a week/ fortnight you cover each muscle group.

Resistance training sometimes gets pushed to one side, especially in the female market where the focus is so strongly on weight loss. I have had many a client grumble about including resistance exercises in their programme as they have an irrational fear that, within a couple of weeks, they will have muscles to rival the incredible hulk! Resistance training with the ball, using just your body weight, or some light hand weights, will certainly not give you big bulky muscles. In fact, quite the opposite happens, the ball encourages long lean muscles, a strong centre and great posture – think of the poise of a dancer.

As well as giving us tone, strength and definition, resistance training has many other benefits. It has a lot to offer to a weight loss programme, as not only do the exercises burn calories, but having more muscle tone increases your metabolic rate, so you will continue to burn extra calories long after your workout has finished. Training with weight bearing exercises also slows down the natural process of loss of bone strength and density. It has been

proven to greatly reduce our chances of suffering from the debilitating condition of osteoporosis later in life. Various studies have also proven that resistance training can help to reduce blood pressure and lower blood cholesterol levels.

There are endless opportunities to adapt exercises to suit your needs. Don't be afraid to adjust an exercise slightly if it doesn't suit your body, and quite often it is possible to use the ball for extra support when needed. On the flip side, don't fall into the trap of always doing the exercises that you find the easiest! Try to select some you find more challenging as these will probably do you the most good!

When using the ball you will find that you can work every muscle in your body, some of which you may even be discovering for the first time. You will find it easier to isolate the larger muscle groups than on the traditional flat surface of the floor or bench and you will automatically be working the small stabiliser muscles to keep you balanced on the ball, giving you stronger, less injury-prone joints.

Remember, though, that you are working on an unstable surface that is constantly challenging your centre of gravity. The key is to always keep your movement under conscious control. When you work too fast you lose control of the movement and momentum takes over. This will mean that, driven by momentum and not your muscles, the exercise will be much less effective and you will be at much greater risk of injury or losing balance. A good test of control is making sure you can stop at any point in each exercise.

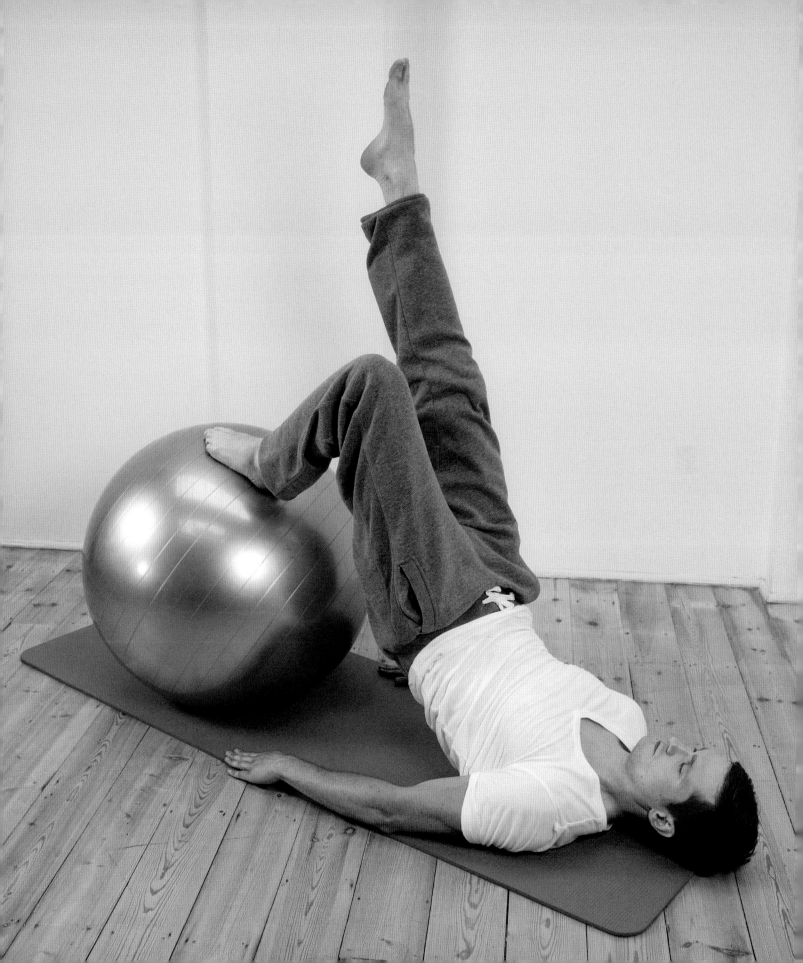

UPPER BODY EXERCISES

BALL FRONT RAISES

? **WHAT FOR?** To tone and strengthen the muscles in the shoulders.

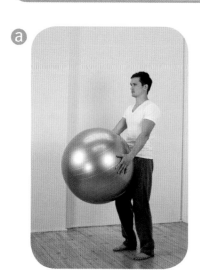
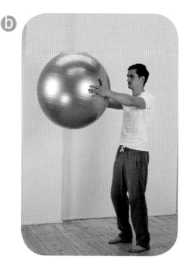
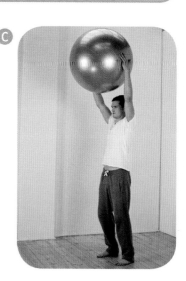

1 **a** Start standing with your feet hip width apart, knees slightly relaxed, core contracted, holding the ball in both hands.

2 Raise your arms first up to shoulder height, pausing briefly here, **b** then above your head. **c**

3 Now slowly lower your arms all the way back down to your starting position.

TIPS

- Keep the elbows relaxed – don't lock the joint.
- Avoid leaning your weight backwards as the arms lift, contracting your core will ensure this doesn't happen.
- Stay in control of the movement. Don't be tempted to throw the arms up quickly, especially when the ball starts to feel heavy!

HOOVER

 WHAT FOR? To strengthen the muscles in the lower back. You will also be recruiting all of those deep stabiliser muscles to keep you balanced on the ball.

1 Start on your hands and knees over the ball. Walk yourself out onto your hands until the ball is underneath your thighs. When you are there, still maintaining neutral spine position, lower yourself down onto your elbows and link your fingers so that your forearms are in a triangle shape. Activate your abdominal contraction and make sure that you body is in a straight diagonal line from your shoulders to your toes.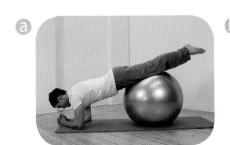

2 Keeping the straight diagonal line throughout, slowly roll yourself forwards so that you are lowering your nose over your hands towards the floor in front. **ⓑ**

3 Now, keeping control, roll yourself back to your starting position.

4 Repeat the movement 12–15 times.

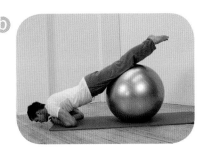

 INCREASE THE LEVEL

1 Start on your hand and knees over the ball as before. This time as you walk out on the ball, walk further, stopping when the ball is underneath the lower legs. Come down onto your elbows and link your fingers as before.

2 Repeat steps 2–4 as before.

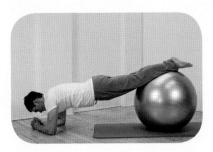

TIPS

- Your core contraction will enable you to maintain the diagonal position. Imagine you are a plank of wood that does not bend or sag in the middle.
- Only lower as far over as you feel comfortable with. Allow yourself to build up over time if you find this tough on the upper body initially.
- Keep the movement steady and controlled.
- Try to coordinate your breathing. Breathe out as you roll forwards and breathe in as you return to your starting position.

SWIMMING

? WHAT FOR? To strengthen the muscles in the lower back. You will also be recruiting all of those deep stabiliser muscles to keep you balanced on the ball.

1 **ⓐ** Start on your hands and knees over the ball.

2 **ⓑ** Now extend your legs and place your hands onto the ball, finding your balance in this position.

3 Start your swimming by using your right arm in a breast stroke motion. Push the arm forwards as you lower the upper body over the ball **ⓒ** and then pull the arm all the way around to your side as you extend the upper body up, coming taller than the ball **ⓓ**

4 Take 12–15 repetitions, alternating arms

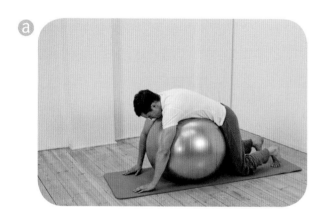

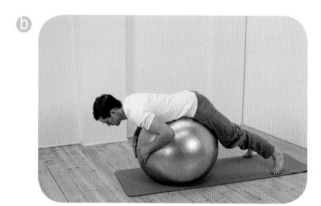

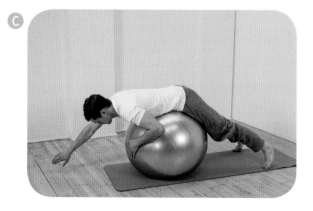

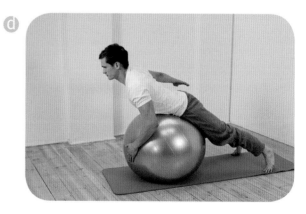

1 Repeat steps 1 and 2 above.
2 When swimming in step 3, use both arms in a breaststroke motion simultaneously. **ⓔ ⓕ**
3 Step 4 as before.

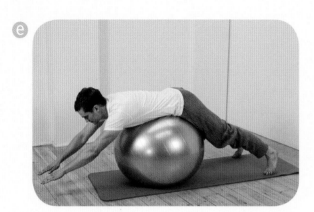

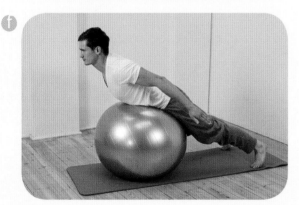

TIPS

- When swimming with one arm, keep your other arm placed on the ball for support and balance.
- When extending the upper body, aim for a straight diagonal line between your head and feet. Try not to over extend as this will put pressure on the lower back.
- If you find this exercise too difficult, try keeping your knees on the floor until you build up a bit more strength in the lower back.

PRESS UPS

? WHAT FOR? To strengthen and tone the muscles in the chest, shoulders and triceps. This is also a great exercise for testing your neutral spine position and core contraction. Much more versatile than the traditional press up on the floor!

 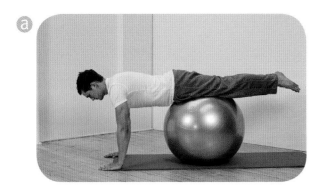

1 Start on your hands and knees over the ball. Walk yourself out forwards onto your hands and keep walking, allowing the ball to roll down your legs. Stop when the ball is underneath your thighs. Ensure that your hands are directly under your shoulders and your core contraction is activated maintaining your neutral spine position. **a**

2 Bend your arms, lowering your nose towards the floor. Keep your focus down to the floor and make sure that your back does not sag in the middle. **b**

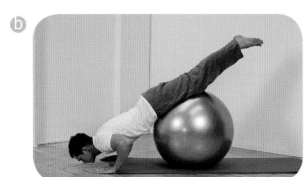

3 Extend your elbows again pushing into the floor through the heel of your hands. **c**

4 Repeat 12–15 times. Walk your hands back in until you come onto your hands and knees over the ball.

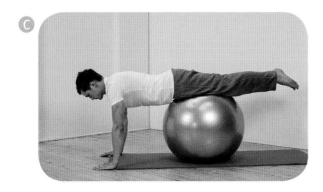

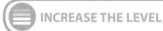
1   Repeat step 1 as before but continue walking out on your ball until it is underneath your lower leg. The further you walk out, the harder this exercise will become. Make sure that you only walk out as far as you can maintain neutral position in your spine. **d**

2   Repeat steps 2–4 as before.

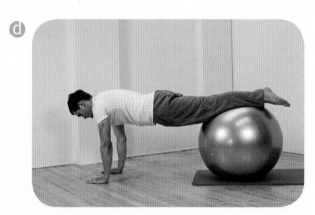

Advanced level

You can also try walking out even further on the ball until the ball is underneath the balls of your feet. **e** This is a very advanced exercise so only attempt it when you have built up enough strength to stabilise the spine in this position.

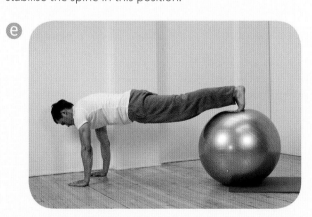

TIPS

- Your shoulders should be directly over your wrists at all times throughout the exercise. Don't allow yourself to roll backwards on the ball.

- Keep your elbows slightly softened when extended, don't lock the joint.

- Your spine must stay supported by your core contraction. Do not start sagging in the lower back. This will put a lot of pressure on your spine and could potentially cause injury. If you feel this happening, walk yourself back onto your ball a bit until you feel happy that you can maintain neutral spine position.

- Your body should remain strong and stable as a whole unit throughout.

- Keep your focus down to the floor. This will ensure that your head stays in line with the rest of the spine.

- Coordinate your breathing. Breathe in as you lower and out as you push up.

TRICEP DIPS

1 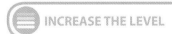 Start sitting on the floor with your legs placed on top of your ball, hands resting on the floor behind you with your fingers pointing in towards your body. Sit up tall in this position and lean your weight back into your arms.

2 Now slowly bend your elbows whilst keeping your spine straight.

3 Then extend again coming back to your starting position.

4 Take 12–15 repetitions.

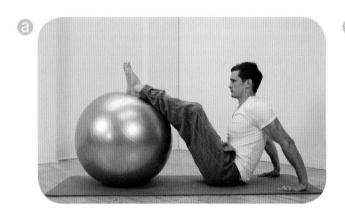

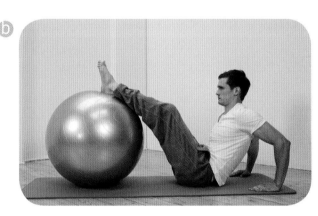

INCREASE THE LEVEL

1 Start sitting as before in step 1, but this time lift your bottom off the floor.

2 Repeat steps 2–4 as before, keeping your bottom off the floor.

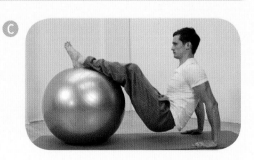

ADVANCED LEVEL

1 **d** Start seated on the front of the ball with your hands resting on the ball behind you, fingers pointing in towards your body.
2 **e** Take your weight onto your arms and lift your bottom off the ball.
3 **f** Slowly bend your elbows, keeping your balance.
4 Extend the elbows again trying to keep the wrists and arms stabilised throughout.
5 Take 8–10 repetitions.

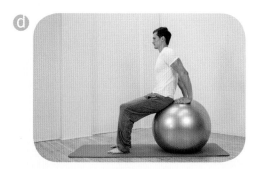

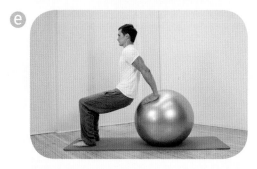

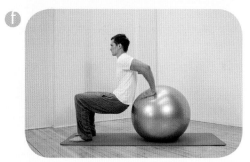

TIPS

- Try to keep the body stabilised in position throughout. The only moving body part should be the elbow.
- Keep your spine extended throughout. It is tempting to round the back as the elbows bend, so focus on the lengthening the spine.
- Build up slowly through the levels, don't be tempted to go for the advanced level until you have built up enough strength in the upper body to stabilise the joints.

LOWER BODY EXERCISES

WALL SQUATS

? WHAT FOR? To tone and shape the legs and buttocks.

1 **a** Place the ball in the small of your back and allow it to support you as you lean your weight into the wall. Walk your feet out so they are about a stride in front of your body.

2 **b** Bend your knees, allowing the ball to roll up your spine until your thighs are parallel with the floor.

3 Now straighten your legs, returning to your start position.

4 Repeat the exercise 10–15 times.

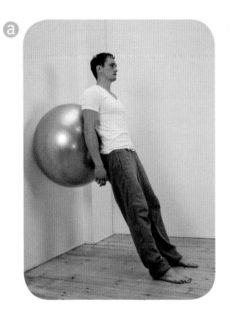

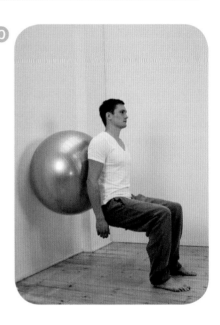

1 Start as before in step 1.
2 Again bend your knees, allowing the ball to roll up your spine until your thighs are parallel with the floor.
3 ⓒ Lift your heels off the floor.
4 ⓓ Straighten your legs while keeping your heels lifted.
5 Lower your heels back to the floor.
6 Repeat the exercise 10–15 times.

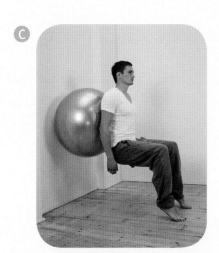

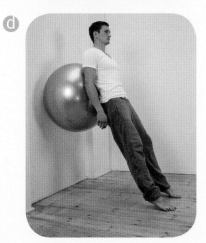

TIPS

- When you are in the squat position, you should still be able to see your toes over your knees. If you can't, you need to walk your feet further away from the wall when in your starting position.
- Keeping your core muscles engaged throughout the exercise will help you stay balanced.
- If you would like to make the exercise a little easier while you build strength in your legs, try taking a smaller squat to begin with.

BALL SQUATS

 WHAT FOR? To tone and shape the legs and buttocks. The rolling action of the ball enables us to recreate the leg press action you may have seen used on machines in the gym.

1 Start sitting on the ball. Walk yourself out, allowing the ball to roll up your spine and lying yourself back onto the ball. Keep walking until the ball is underneath your shoulder blades and the back of your head is resting on the ball. Check that your knees are directly over your ankles, and your hips are lifted to the same height as your knees. Place your hands across your chest. ⓐ

2 ⓑ Now lower your hips towards the floor, sitting down into a squat allowing the ball to roll with you.

3 Next push your heels into the floor rolling the ball back again and lifting the hips as you return to your starting position. Repeat the movement 10–15 times.

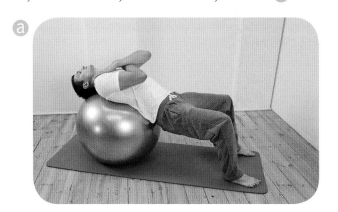

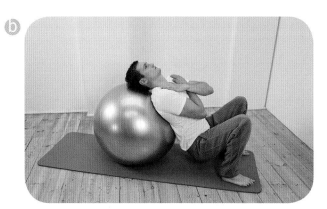

 INCREASE THE LEVEL

1 Repeat steps 1 and 2 as before.
2 This time, as you push back into your starting position, raise one of your feet a few inches off the floor so you are balancing on the other leg.
3 As you lower back into the squat place both feet back on the floor, and next time you push back, lift the other leg off the floor.
4 Repeat 10–15 times alternating legs. When finished slowly walk yourself back up to a seated position.

TIPS

- Make sure that your knees stay directly over your ankles at all times
- Keep your head relaxed back on the ball to avoid any tension in the neck.
- Keep the movement controlled throughout – never bounce.

PRONE BOTTOM SQUEEZES

? **WHAT FOR?** To increase tone and definition of the bottom.

1   Start on your hands and knees over the ball. Now push your weight forwards so that you can rest your elbows on the floor, linking your fingers together and resting your forehead on your hands. Extend the legs behind you so the balls of the feet are resting on the floor and turn the legs out so that the knees and feet are pointing out at a 45-degree angle. **a**

2   **b** Lift the legs off the floor until you are in a straight diagonal line from your head to feet.

3   Take small bounces with the legs so they lower a few inches, and then lift again as you squeeze the muscles in the bottom hard.

4   Repeat 20–30 squeezes then rest.

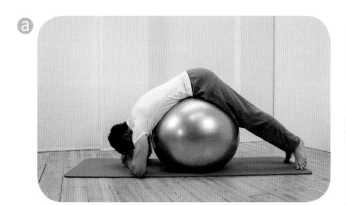

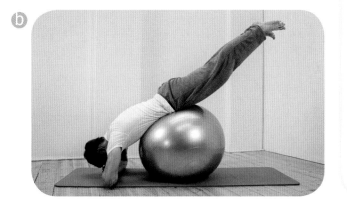

TIPS

- The movement in the legs should be happening as a result of the muscles in the bottom being squeezed. Try to make sure that you are not just moving the legs up and down.
- Keep the rest of the body stabilised throughout to avoid losing balance on the ball.
- You should feel this in the bottom and the backs of your legs. If you feel it at all in the lower back then take your weight a little further forwards onto your arms.

SIDE LYING ABDUCTOR LIFTS

? **WHAT FOR?** To tone and strengthen the muscles of the outer thigh.

1 **a** Start kneeling with the ball on your right side.

2 **b** Reach your right arm over the ball placing it on the floor, and extend your left leg out to the side. Keep your hips and shoulders square on to the front. Rest your left hand on top of the ball to keep it steady.

3 **c** Lift your left leg up to the side until it is level with your hip.

4 Now slowly lower the leg back down to your starting position, keeping it a few inches off the floor.

5 Repeat 10–15 times, and then again on the other side.

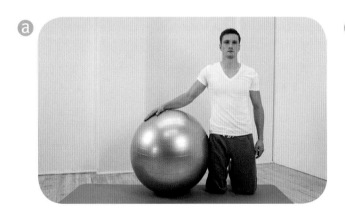

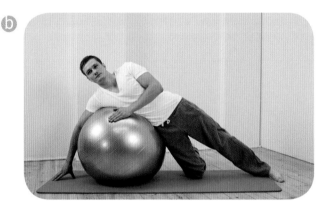

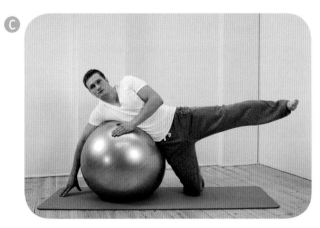

TIPS

- This should be a slow, controlled lifting and lowering movement, not a kick.
- If you feel any tension in your neck, try bending your underneath arm and resting your head on your hand.
- Coordinate your breathing. Breathe in as you raise your leg and breathe out as you lower.

SIDE LYING ADDUCTOR LIFTS

? WHAT FOR? To tone and strengthen the muscles of the inner thigh.

1 **a** Start kneeling with the ball on your right side.

2 **b** Reach your right arm over the ball placing it on the floor. Bend your left leg and place the foot on the floor in front of you and extend your right leg underneath the left. Keep your hips and shoulders square on to the front. Place your left hand on the ball for support.

3 **c** Lift the right leg a few inches off the floor.

4 Then lower the leg back down to your starting position.

5 Repeat the lifts 10–15 times, moving quite quickly.

a

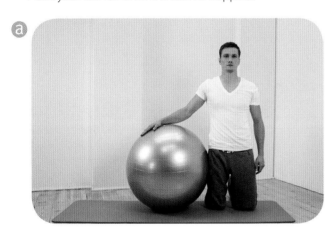

b

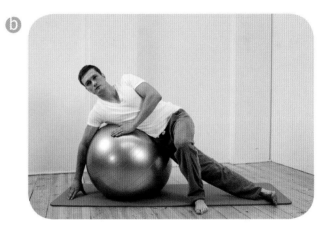

c

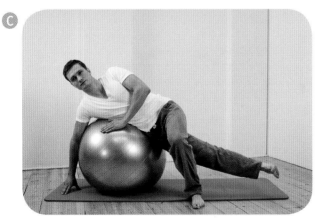

TIPS

- Don't try and lift the underneath leg too high, a small movement is enough.
- Squeeze the inner thigh muscles as you lift.
- If you feel any tension in your neck, try bending your underneath arm and resting your head on your hand.

LEG BEATS

? WHAT FOR? To tone and define the muscles in the backs of the legs and the bottom. This follows nicely on from the previous two exercises if you would like a little routine for the bottom area!

1 Start on your hands and knees over the ball. Now push your weight forwards so that you can rest your elbows on the floor, linking your fingers together and resting your forehead on your hands. Extend the legs behind you so the balls of the feet are resting on the floor and turn the legs out so that the knees and feet are pointing out at a 45-degree angle.

2 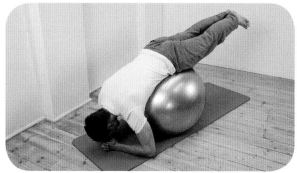 Lift your legs off the floor behind you until your feet are slightly higher than your hips and hold here.

3 Now beat your heels together in a small movement, squeezing the bottom throughout.

4 Beat 30–50 times then relax.

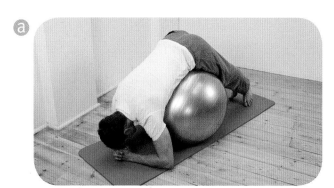

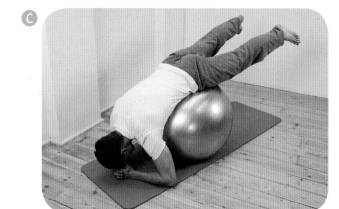

TIPS

- Keep your legs lifted above hip height as you beat the heels together.
- If you feel this at all in the lower back, try taking your weight a little further forward onto your arms.
- Breathe steadily throughout, don't hold your breath!

ADDUCTOR SQUEEZES

? WHAT FOR? To tone and strengthen the muscles of the inner thigh.

1 Start lying on your back with your knees bent, feet flat on the floor, your arms relaxed by your sides and the ball held between your knees.

2 Squeeze the ball as hard as you can for a couple of seconds and then rest for a couple of seconds.

3 Repeat the squeezes 25–30 times.

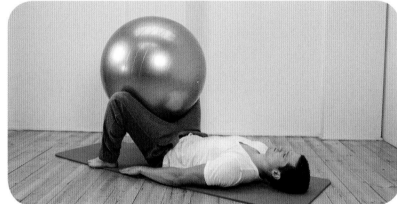

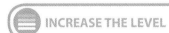 **INCREASE THE LEVEL**

1 Start lying on your back, this time place the ball between your ankles and extend your legs into the air so that your ankles are directly above your hips. Keep your arms relaxed by your sides.

2 Repeat steps 2 and 3 as before.

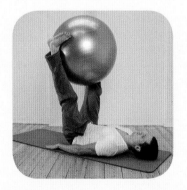

TIPS

- Imagine you are trying to burst your ball as you squeeze!
- Keep your core contraction in place to prevent the back from arching as you squeeze.
- Try to keep breathing throughout the exercise; don't hold your breath.
- If you are trying a more difficult level, make sure your ankles stay above your hips. Avoid allowing them to lower as you get tired, as this will apply pressure to the lower back.

HAMSTRING CURLS

 WHAT FOR? To tone and strengthen the back of the legs and the bottom. This one takes a bit of getting used to, so don't worry if you find it difficult to start with!

1 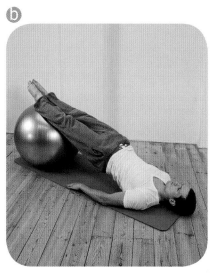 Start lying on the floor with your arms by your sides. Place your feet on the ball and walk it away from you until your legs are straight.

2 Lift your hips off the floor by curling up through the spine until your body is in a straight diagonal line from your feet to your shoulders.

3 Now bend your knees, rolling your heels in to your bottom. Keep the straight diagonal line between your knees and your bottom by lifting the hips higher as you roll the ball in.

4 Now slowly roll the ball back out to your starting position. Repeat 10–12 times.

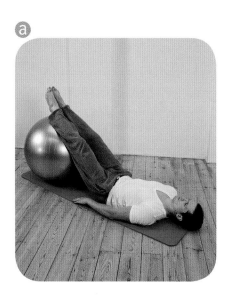

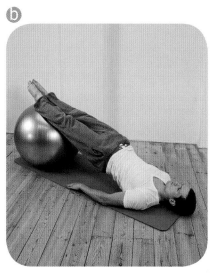

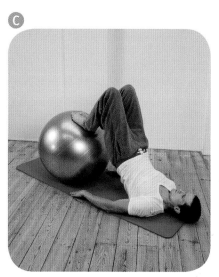

1 Repeat steps 1 and 2 as before.
2 **d** Raise your right leg a few inches above the ball.
3 **e** Roll the ball in and out as before with just your left leg, while keeping the right one extended.

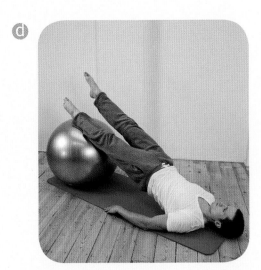

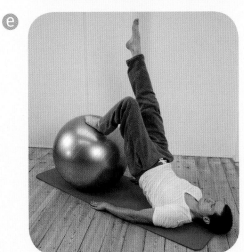

TIPS

- When rolling the ball in, use your heels to push into the ball.
- Keeping your feet hip width apart on the ball will give you a wider base of support, making it a little easier to balance.
- Make sure you are comfortable with the two-leg version before moving on to the one-leg curl.
- Coordinate your breathing. Breathe in as you roll your legs in, and breathe out as you extend them.

ABDOMINAL EXERCISES

TRUNK CURLS

> **?** **WHAT FOR?** To strengthen and tone the abdominal muscles. This is traditional curls on an unstable surface, great for that six-pack!

1 **a** Start seated on your ball with your feet hip width apart, knees directly over ankles and your hands placed lightly on the ball.

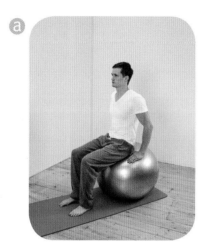

2 **b** Slowly walk your feet forwards, allowing yourself to lie back into the ball as it rolls up your spine. Stop when the ball is underneath your lower back, making sure your knees are still directly over your ankles. Your shoulders should be higher than your knees, at about a 45-degree incline position.

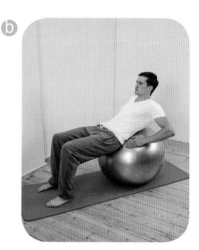

3 **c** Place your hands across your chest. Activate your core contraction.

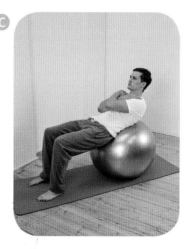

4 **d** Curl the upper body, drawing the ribcage towards the hips. When you have curled up as far as is comfortable, slowly control the movement back down to your starting position.

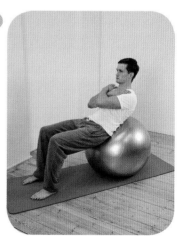

5 Repeat the curl 12–15 times.

INCREASE THE LEVEL

1 Repeat steps 1 and 2 as before.
2 This time perform the curls with the hands lightly touching the temples, or if you want to make it even more challenging, extend your arms above your head.

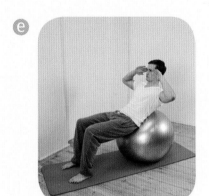

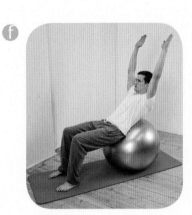

Advanced level

1 Repeat steps 1 and 2 as before.
2 Once you are in the incline position, take two steps back in towards your ball so that more of your body is suspended over the back of the ball. This is called the tabletop position; your hips, knees and shoulders should all be the same level so you look flat like a table. Choose your hand position from the options in the previous level.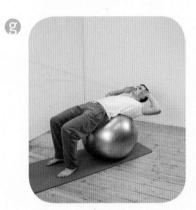
3. Take 12–15 curls in this position.

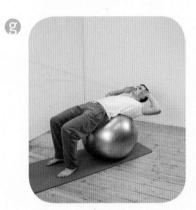

TIPS

- To ensure that you are staying in control of the movement try counting 3 seconds as you lift and 3 seconds as you lower.
- If your hands are placed on your temples, don't be tempted to pull on the head as you lift up.
- Make sure the torso is curling, rather than the ball rolling. The ball should stay very still throughout.
- When in the lowering phase of the exercise, don't lower down too far allowing the spine to overarch.
- Try coordinating your breathing with the movement. Breathe out as you lift and breathe in as you lower down.

OBLIQUE CURLS AGAINST THE WALL

? WHAT FOR? To strengthen and tone the abdominal and oblique muscles. You can also do the Trunk Curls (page 72) in this position.

1 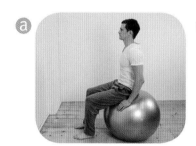 Start seated on your ball just over a leg's length away from a clear, flat wall. Have your feet hip width apart and knees directly over your hips. Place your hands lightly on the ball.

2 ⓑ Slowly walk your feet forwards, allowing yourself to lie back into the ball as it rolls up your spine. Stop when the ball is underneath your lower back. Place your feet on the wall in front of you at least hip width apart, shins parallel with the floor. Place your hands either on your temples or across your chest as described in the previous exercise.

3 ⓒ Curl your upper body as far as you feel comfortable. Keeping the curl in place, twist your body to look to the left side, ⓓ then twist back to the centre ⓔ and lower back down. ⓕ Don't bend backwards over the ball further than your neutral spine position, and try not to allow any tension in your neck.

4 Repeat 12–15 times alternating sides.

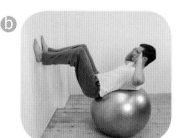
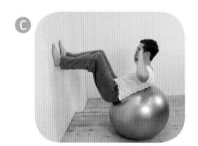
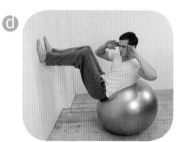
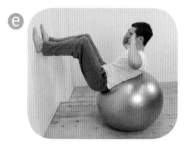
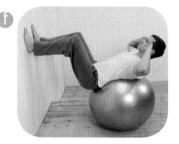

 INCREASE THE LEVEL

1 Repeat steps 1 and 2 as before.
2 This time you are going to circle with the upper body.
3 Lift up to the centre to start.
   Circle around to the right.
   Circle down as you come to the centre.
   Circle around to the left.
   Lift back up to the centre to finish.
4 Repeat the circles 6–8 times alternating sides.

SCISSOR LEG REVERSE CURLS

? WHAT FOR? To tone and strengthen the muscles of the lower abdomen. Great for that little bulge that us ladies find hard to shift.

1 **a** Start lying on the floor with the ball gripped between your legs in a scissor position, the right leg in front of the ball, the left leg behind. Have your arms relaxed by your sides.

2 **b** Curl your knees in towards your shoulders, allowing your bottom to lift off the floor a few inches.

3 Now slowly lower back to your starting position.

4 Repeat the curls 10–15 times, then change sides.

a

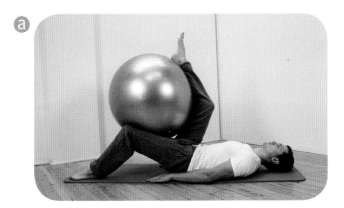

b

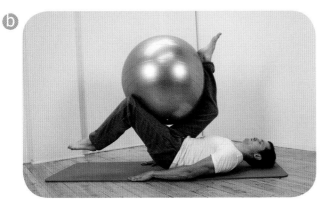

TIPS

- Make sure that the movement is coming from the abdominal muscles not from pushing your hands against the floor. If you can't help but use your hands, lightly place them across your chest to take temptation out of the way!
- This movement is more of a squeeze than a lift and should be slow and controlled. If you allow your legs to start swinging, momentum will take over and the abdominals will do a lot less work.
- Coordinate your breathing with the movement. Breathe out as you lift and breathe in as you lower.

SIDE LYING OBLIQUE CURLS

? WHAT FOR? To tone and strengthen the oblique muscles, really pulling in and defining the waistline.

1 **ⓐ** Start kneeling with the ball by your right side.

2 **ⓑ** Place your left hand onto the ball to stop any movement, then reach your right arm over the top until you're in a side bend. Check that your hips and shoulders are square on to the front.

3 **ⓒ** Extend your top leg out to the side, pushing the foot into the floor to secure yourself. Place your right

hand onto your temple, and keep the left hand lightly touching the top of the ball.

4 **ⓓ** Now slowly lift your upper body sideways off the ball, and then lower back down.

5 Repeat 12–15 times, then change sides.

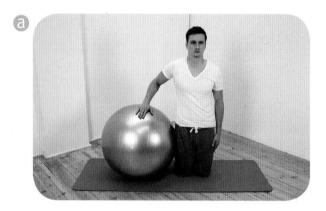
ⓐ

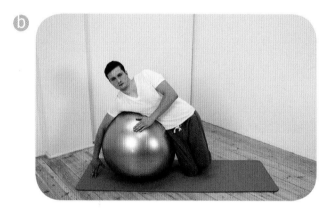
ⓑ

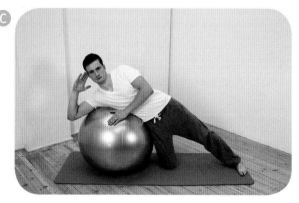
ⓒ

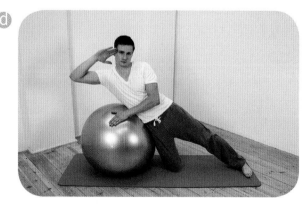
ⓓ

1 Repeat steps 1–2 as before.
2 This time extend your top leg out to the side as before then place your fingers either on your temples **e** or to make it even more of a challenge, extend your arms overhead. **f**
3 Repeat steps 4–5 as before.

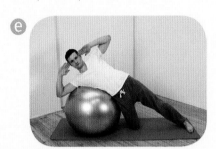

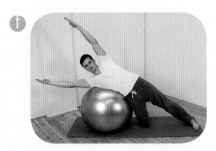

Advanced level

1 Repeat steps 1 and 2 as before.
2 This time bend your top leg and place the foot on the floor in front of your hip. Then extend your bottom leg underneath. **g**
3 Choose which arm position you will use as described in the previous two levels.
4 Repeat the exercise in this position as before.
5 If you would like to progress the leg position even further try the scissor position. Extend your top leg out to the side, taking it slightly forwards of the line of the body. Then extend your bottom leg as well, taking it slightly behind the line of the body. In this position you may need to place your hip a little further onto the ball than before. Place either the underneath hand to the temple keeping the top hand on the ball for support, or both hands to temples if you want more of a challenge. **h**

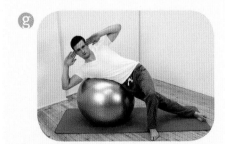

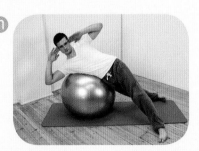

TIPS

- At first you may find it difficult to balance in the side lying positions, or find that your feet keep slipping out from underneath you. If this happens try the exercise near a wall and push your supporting leg(s) against the wall to hold you in position.
- Gradually work your way up through the levels after you are confident you can keep stability throughout the body and stay balanced on the ball.
- As your body lifts make sure you stay square to the front. Don't allow the shoulders to twist outwards.
- Don't try to lift too high to start with. Once your body gets used to the exercise and builds strength you will be able to lift higher.
- Try to coordinate your breathing with the movement. Breathe out as you lift up and breathe in as you lower back down.

DOUBLE LEG CYCLES

? WHAT FOR? To tone and strengthen the muscles of the lower abdomen.

1 **ⓐ** Start sitting on the floor with the ball gripped between your ankles. Lower yourself down so that you are resting your weight onto your elbows, and bend your knees in to your chest.

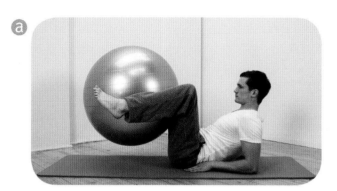

2 **ⓑ** Extend your legs out to a 45-degree angle, then continue in a circle allowing the legs to lift up to a vertical position **ⓒ** then bend back in to the starting position. **ⓐ**

3 Take 8–10 circles.

4 Now reverse the movement, extending the legs to a vertical position first **ⓒ**, lowering them down to a 45-degree angle **ⓑ** and then bending them back in to your starting position. **ⓐ**

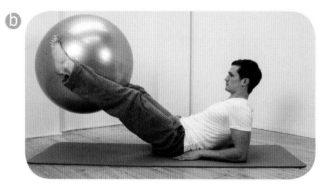

TIPS

- Your core contraction is really important here to stop your spine arching when the legs are extended out to a 45-degree angle. If you feel your back is starting to arch, lift the legs into a higher position where you feel you can maintain stability in the lower back.
- Really focus on pulling in the lower abdominal muscles as you extend the legs out.

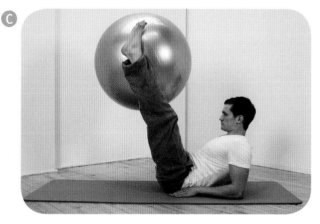

KNEELING BALL ROLLS

? **WHAT FOR?** To strengthen and tone the abdominals and the upper body.

1 **a** Start kneeling, sitting back onto your heels. Link your fingers together and place your hands on the ball, level with your chest.

2 **b** Start to roll the ball forwards, coming up onto your knees and allowing the ball to roll up your forearms. Keep going until your body is in a straight diagonal line from your knees to your shoulders and your elbows are resting on the ball.

3 Roll the ball back in, sitting yourself down again into your starting position.

4 Repeat 8–10 times.

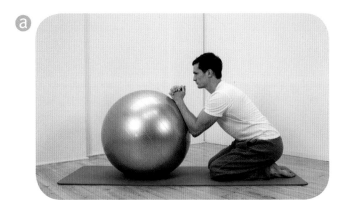

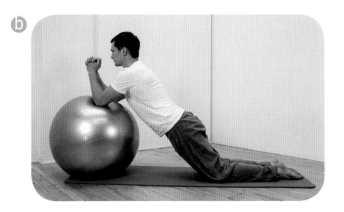

TIPS

- Do not collapse in the middle and allow your spine to arch. It is by maintaining your core contraction throughout that your spine will stay supported. If you cannot maintain the position of the spine take smaller rolls until you have built up more core strength.
- The ball should only be coming into contact with the arms throughout this exercise. Make sure that your upper body is not resting on the ball.
- Coordinate your breathing with the movement. Breathe out as you roll out, and breathe in as you return.

FULL BODY INTEGRATION

BALL PLANK

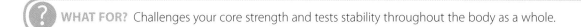

? WHAT FOR? Challenges your core strength and tests stability throughout the body as a whole.

1 **ⓐ** Start kneeling down in front of the ball with your forearms placed on the ball, fists clenched.

2 **ⓑ** Lower your body down so your shoulders are resting on your fists, then extend your legs out behind you so the balls of the feet are pushing into the floor.

3 Contract your core, and maintain neutral spine as you hold this position for 20–30 seconds, or as long as you feel able.

TIPS

- The core contraction enables you to maintain neutral spine position so you don't sag in the middle, putting pressure on the spine.
- Remember to breathe; don't hold your breath.

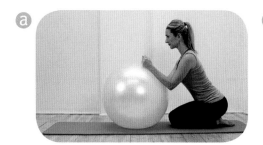

INCREASE THE LEVEL

1 Start kneeling down in front of your ball, with your fingers linked together and your forearms placed on the ball, elbows shoulder width apart. **ⓒ**

2 Extend your legs behind you, pushing the balls of the feet into the floor. **ⓓ**

3 Repeat step 3 as before.

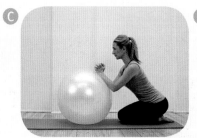

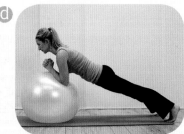

PELVIC LIFTS

 WHAT FOR? To mobilise the spine and to practise core strength and stability, integrating the body as a whole. This exercise is actually also a wonderful massage around the spine.

1 Start lying on the floor with your arms relaxed by your sides. Place the ball underneath your legs so that your calves are resting against the ball.

2 Slowly peel the hips and spine away from the floor, lifting one vertebra at a time until the pelvis is lifted.

There should be a straight diagonal line from your shoulders to your feet.

3 Curl back down again through the spine, working through each vertebra until your hips have returned to the starting position.

4 Repeat the lifts 6–8 times.

TIPS

- This exercise should be executed slowly and thoughtfully, really being aware of each vertebra as you roll up and down through the spine.
- Your core contraction is what will keep you balanced on the ball throughout this exercise, so make sure it is in place before you start.
- Try and keep your arms relaxed on the floor next to you. It is very tempting to try and hold on to the floor for balance.
- Coordinate your breathing with the movement. Breathe out as your pelvis lifts up and breathe in as you lower.

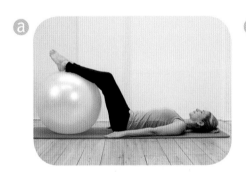

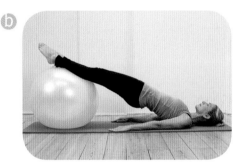

INCREASE THE LEVEL

1 Start lying on the floor with your arms relaxed by your sides. This time place the ball underneath your legs so that your heels are resting on the ball.

2 Repeat steps 2 to 4 as before.

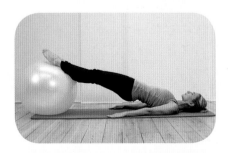

KNEELING BALANCE

 WHAT FOR? This is your ultimate balance challenge on the ball; you will need to recruit all of those stability muscles to keep you balanced and steady. Falling off is a real possibility, but practise makes perfect!

TIPS

- When sitting back onto your heels, make sure that your knees are as wide apart as you are able on the ball. This will give you a wider base of support making it a little easier to balance.
- Focus on a fixed object throughout the exercise to aid your balance and concentration.
- Only take the exercise as far as you feel comfortable. Your balance will quickly improve if you regularly work with the ball, so try again in a few weeks if you don't feel ready for this exercise now.
- Make sure that there is nothing around you that will cause injury if you do fall off the ball!

1 **a** Start on your hands and knees over the ball.

2 **b** Walk yourself out onto your hands allowing the ball to roll down your legs. Stop when the ball is underneath your thighs.

3 **c** Bend your knees, allowing the ball to roll in, and then sit back onto your heels, still with your hands on the floor.

4 **d** Try having a little test here to see if you can place one of your hands onto the ball, and then the other in turn.

5 **e** Try and take both hands and place them on the ball. Use your hands to help stabilise the ball by pushing and pulling on it when necessary.

6 **f** If you feel you are on balance and can take this to the next stage then try taking your hands completely off the ball and rising up onto your knees. Your arms should be pointing out to the sides of the room to help you balance.

7 Balance for as long as you feel able. Reverse the steps to bring yourself off the ball again.

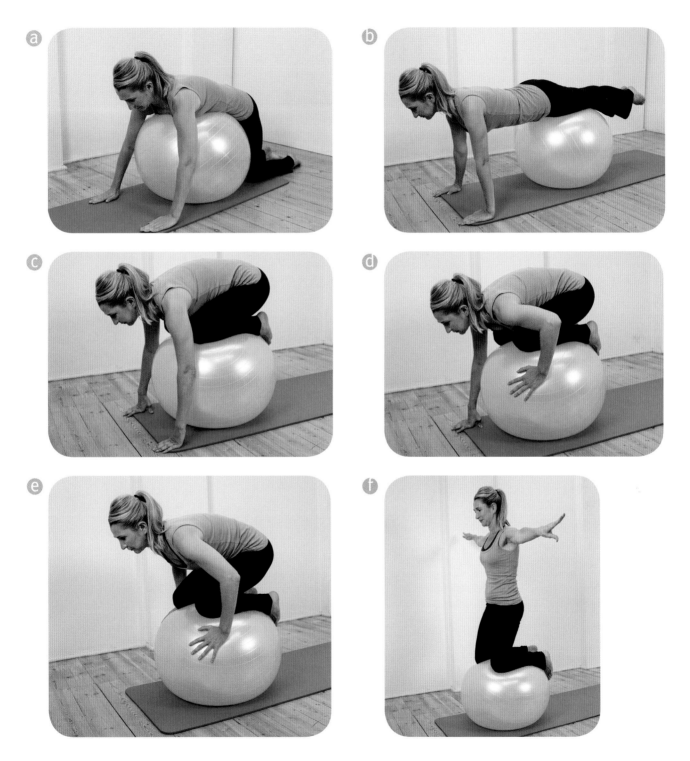

USING HAND WEIGHTS WITH THE BALL

For the following exercises you are going to need a set of hand weights. Don't worry if you don't have any, they are very easy and cheap to make yourself. See below for making your weights.

In most cases with the ball you can recreate exercises performed on traditional weights equipment without any equipment at all, and there is certainly an alternative exercise for each body part you may normally target with weights or resistance equipment. However there is another benefit to using the ball as a support while you perform more traditional hand weights exercises.

The ball is of course unstable, so you are not only working the target muscle group during each of the exercises, but you are also working all of those deep stabiliser muscles throughout your core and your legs to keep you balanced. It's a bit like two or even three exercises for the price of one… and we all like a bargain!

MAKING YOUR WEIGHTS

○ Take two plastic drinks bottles (large ones are better, you can make them heavier if necessary).

○ Fill them with the amount of water you would like. You can use a set of kitchen scales to weigh your weight – I would suggest starting with a 2lb or 3lb weight and seeing how you get on.

○ Adjust your weights by increasing/decreasing the amount of water. You may find for some exercises you need a lighter weight than for others.

○ Make sure when performing each exercise that your weight is heavy enough to make you feel like you are tiring for the last few repetitions, but not so heavy that you are struggling after just a few!

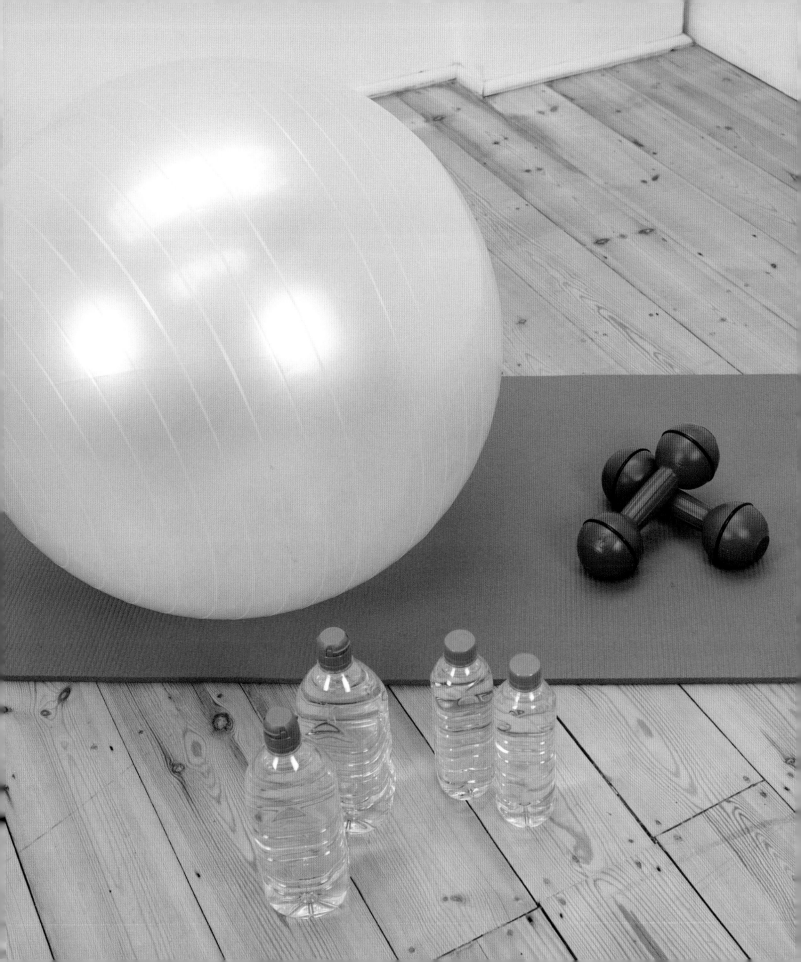

CHEST PRESS

 WHAT FOR? To strengthen and tone the muscles in the chest and the backs of the arms. You will also have to work hard to keep yourself balanced on the ball throughout.

1 Start seated on the ball, holding your weights in close to your torso.

2 **b** Walk your feet out, allowing the ball to roll up your spine and lying yourself back onto the ball. Keep walking until the ball is resting underneath your shoulder blades and rest your head onto the ball. Your hips should be level with your knees and your knees directly over your ankles. Place your weights so that they are directly over your shoulders.

3 **c** Extend your arms forwards so that your weights are level with your chest. Then bend your elbows again bringing your weights back to the starting position.

5 Take 10–15 repetitions.

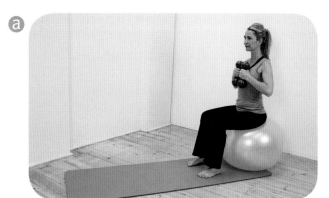

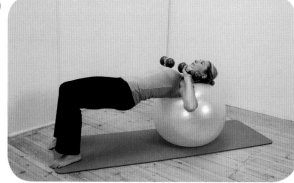

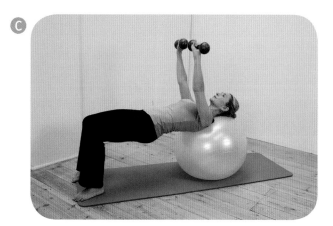

TIPS

- Keep the weights in line with your chest throughout.
- When the arms are extended be careful not to lock your elbows as this will apply excess pressure to the joint.
- Keep each repetition steady and controlled.
- Coordinate your breathing. Breathe out as your arms extend, and breathe in as you lower.

FLIES

? WHAT FOR? To tone and strengthen the muscles in your chest and shoulders. This is another traditional exercise usually performed on a stable bench in the gym.

1 **a** Start seated on the ball, holding your weights in close to your torso.

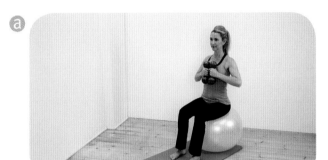

2 **b** Walk your feet out, allowing the ball to roll up your spine and lying yourself back onto the ball. Keep walking until the ball is resting underneath your shoulder blades and rest your head on the ball. Your hips should be level with your knees and your knees directly over your ankles. Extend your arms so that your weights are held above your chest, with your elbows slightly relaxed.

3 **c** Open your arms out from the shoulders, lowering your weights until they are level with your shoulders.

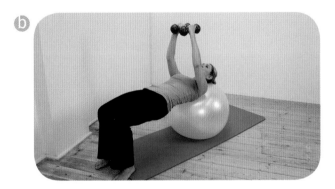

4 Now raise the weights back up into the starting position.

5 Take 10–15 repetitions.

TIPS

- Keep your elbows slightly relaxed so there is a curved shape to your arms throughout. There should be no movement in the elbow joint once in position.
- Focus on your core contraction and neutral spine position. It is easy to allow the back to overarch as the arms lower.
- You should feel a stretch across the chest with each extension.
- Coordinate your breathing. Breathe out as you lower and breathe in as you lift the arms back up.

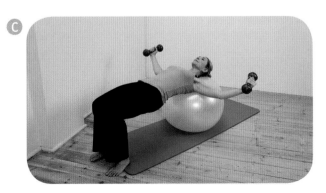

FRONT RAISES

? WHAT FOR? To strengthen and tone the muscles in the shoulders. Great for giving definition to the upper arm.

1 **(a)** Start seated on the ball with your knees bent and feet hip width apart. Hold your weights with your arms relaxed down by your sides.

2 **(b)** Keeping the arms straight, but not locking into the elbows, raise the weights directly up in front of you to shoulder level.

3 Now lower the weights back down to your starting position.

4 Take 10–15 repetitions.

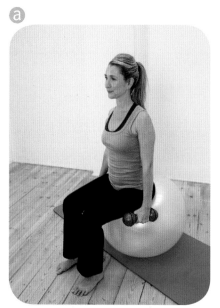

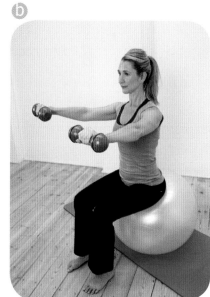

TIPS

- When raising and lowering the arms there should not be any movement in the torso. If you find yourself starting to swing with your upper body, try using a lighter weight.
- Keep the movement steady and controlled throughout.
- Coordinate your breathing. Breathe out as you lift and breathe in as you lower.

BICEP CURLS

? **WHAT FOR?** To tone and strengthen the biceps in the upper arm. Light weights will give a nice definition and shape to the arm.

1 **a** Start seated on the ball, with your knees bent and feet hip width apart. Hold your weights with your arms relaxed down by your sides.

2 **b** Starting with your right arm, bend the elbow, curling the weight up towards the right shoulder.

3 Now lower back to your starting position.

4 Repeat with your left arm.

5 Alternate sides for 10–15 repetitions each side.

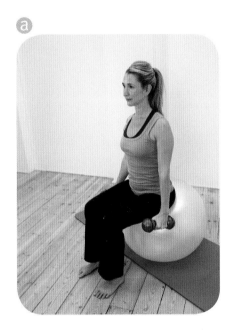

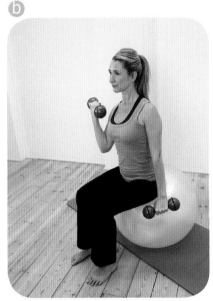

TIPS

- Try to avoid any movement in the torso as the arm moves. Swinging with the body will just make the exercise easier and less effective in targeting the biceps.
- Keep the movement steady and controlled throughout.
- Coordinate your breathing. Breathe out as the arm lifts and breathe in as it lowers.

TRICEP EXTENSIONS

? WHAT FOR? To strengthen and tone the back of the arms. A great bingo wing elimination exercise!

1 **a** Start on your hands and knees over the ball with one weight placed on the floor in front. Pick up the weight with your right hand and keeping your arm in close to your body, lift your elbow behind you.

2 **b** Keeping the elbow lifted, extend the lower part of your arm until your arm is straight.

3 Lower it back down, still keeping the elbow raised.

4 Repeat the extensions 10–15 times then repeat on the other arm.

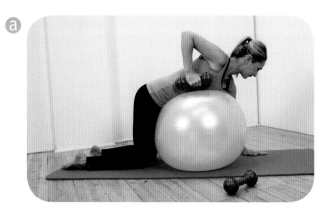

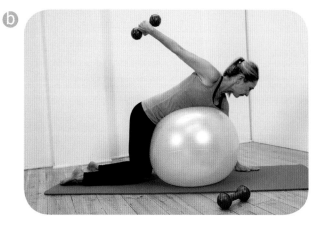

TIPS

- The trick to this exercise is to keep the elbow lifted throughout. There should only be movement from the elbow down, the upper arm should stay fixed throughout.
- Make sure each extension is controlled and doesn't become a swinging movement of the arm.
- Try to coordinate your breathing. Breathe out as you extend and breathe in as the arm lowers.

LYING DOUBLE ARM ROWS

? WHAT FOR? To tone and strengthen the muscles in the upper back.

1 **ⓐ** Start on your hands and knees over the ball with your weights placed on the floor in front of you. Push your weight forwards on the ball slightly so that you are balancing between your hips and the balls of your feet. Pick up your weights and extend your arms out on the floor in front of you.

2 **ⓑ** Bend your arms, keeping them close to your body. Raise the elbows up behind you, squeezing the shoulder blades together as they lift.

3 Slowly lower the arms back to your starting position.

4 Take 10–15 repetitions.

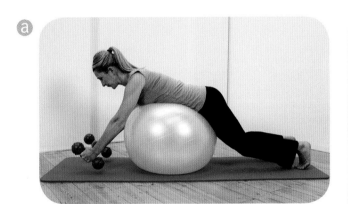

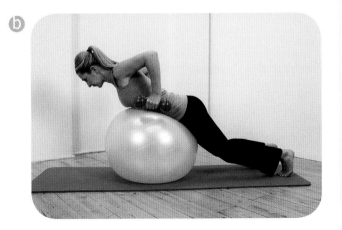

TIPS

- Try to keep your body steady, only allowing movement in the arms.
- Raise the elbows as far as possible in each repetition, without adjusting the body.
- Coordinate your breathing. Breathe out as you lift and breathe in as you lower.

OBLIQUE TWISTS

? WHAT FOR? To tone and strengthen the muscles of both the abdominals and your waist.

1 (a) Start seated on the ball with your knees bent and feet hip width apart. Walk yourself out on the ball, allowing the ball to roll up your spine, stopping when it is underneath your shoulder blades. Your hips should be lifted so they are level with your knees. Pick up one of your weights and hold it in both hands with your arms extended at chest level.

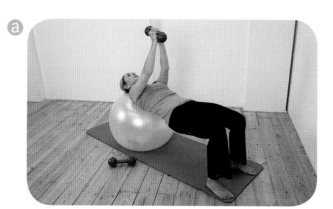

2 Keeping your arms extended, lower your weight down to the right side (b) then in a swinging motion take it all the way over the body to the left side. (c)

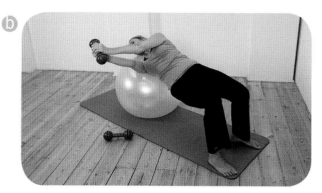

3 Keep swinging from side to side, allowing the upper body to twist slightly with each movement.

4 Take 15–20 repetitions.

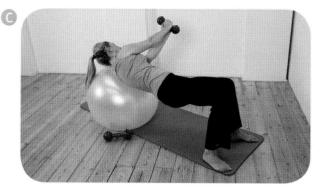

TIPS

- Use the abdominal muscles to initiate each twisting movement rather than just swinging the arms.
- Twist the body as far as you feel able to control the ball and stay balanced.
- Keep the arms extended throughout the movement.
- Keep your focus on your hands, so that your head stays in line with the rest of the spine.

DOUBLE LEG LIFTS

? WHAT FOR? To tone the muscles up the backs of the legs and the bottom. You will also find this works the inner thigh muscles if you grip the weight tight!

1 **ⓐ** Start on your hands and knees over the ball with one of your weights placed on the floor behind you. Come down onto your elbows and link your fingers together, rest your head onto your hands. Now pick up the weight with your legs gripping it between your ankles.

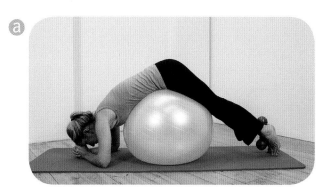

2 **ⓑ** Lift your legs up behind you until they are level with your bottom.

3 **ⓒ** Lower back down to your starting position, keeping the weight lifted a few inches from the floor.

4 Take 10–15 repetitions.

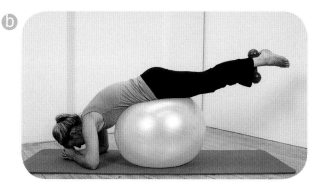

TIPS

- If you are finding it hard to keep the weight gripped between your ankles, try wrapping it in a towel to make it a little less slippery!
- Keep your spine in neutral position as the legs lift; don't allow the lower back to arch.
- Squeeze the bottom on each repetition, making it work a little bit harder.
- Coordinate your breathing. Breathe out as the legs lift and breathe in as they lower.

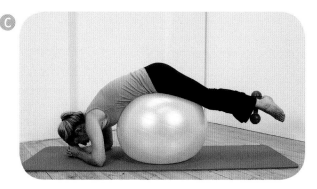

CHAPTER THREE

AEROBICS WITH THE BALL

WHAT IS AEROBIC EXERCISE?

Aerobic is defined as 'with oxygen'. Sometimes called cardiovascular or 'cardio' for short. Aerobic exercise is the type that works up a sweat, causes your breathing rate to increase and makes your heart thump harder. It is any sustained rhythmical activity that uses large muscle groups, meaning the body's need for oxygen is increased.

It can be in the form of running, power walking, cycling, swimming, the stepper or other cardio equipment found in the gym, or it can be in the style of an aerobic class where someone choreographs a routine, in this case with a large rubber ball!

Aerobics is exercise for the heart and lungs as well as your muscles. If aerobically fit, you will manage that steep hill on an afternoon walk without gasping for breath at the top, as well as perhaps keep up with your children running around the park.

Quite often people might have come to aerobic exercise as part of a weight loss programme, whether it was a class at the local centre or a running machine in the gym. Because of the large amount of calories that exercising in this way will burn, it has a very important place alongside a healthy eating plan in the weight loss market.

Aerobic exercise also has a number of other less well known benefits to your mental and physical health. It can increase the size and strength of your heart, reducing your resting heart rate and your chances of heart disease; it can increase the efficiency of your lungs; it is beneficial in improving glucose tolerance and decreasing insulin

resistance which is of course of great benefit for the treatment and prevention of diabetes. On a psychological level it can reduce stress levels, help treat and prevent depression by increasing social interaction, increase the 'feel-good factor' due to the release of endorphins and just generally make people feel better about themselves and their appearance.

AEROBICS WITH THE BALL

Personally I think this is where the ball really comes into its own, as it adds such interest and fun to an aerobic-style workout as well as offering extra challenges not possible without the ball. I haven't met anyone yet who can get through one of my aerobic-style exercise ball classes without breaking into hysterical laughter at some point, and obviously if people are having fun, they are more likely to feel motivated and even more importantly come again. The ball, as well as adding a little of the novelty factor to your workout, also acts as a weight for you to carry, throw and catch, push, circle and bounce around. This introduces an extra challenge to your aerobic exercises that lead to added benefits.

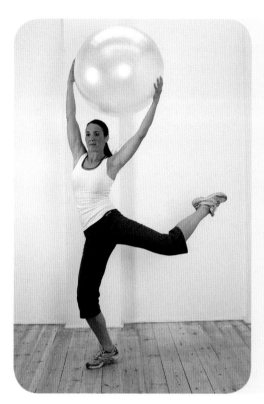

BENEFITS OF AEROBIC EXERCISE AT A GLANCE

○ Increases heart and lung efficiency
○ Burns large amount of calories (30 minutes of moderate intensity aerobics with the ball can burn approximtely 300 calories) so it's great as part of a weight loss programme
○ Increases energy levels
○ Reduces stress and improves mental health due to release of endorphins
○ Reduces blood pressure
○ Lowers resting heart rate
○ Reduces risk of stroke
○ Reduces risk of heart attack
○ Tones and firms all over the body
○ Weight-bearing exercise helps to maintain bone density, reducing the risk of the debilitating condition, osteoporosis, later in life
○ Makes you feel great!

GETTING STARTED

For good cardiovascular fitness it is generally recommended that you should exercise 3–5 times per week for between 30–60 minutes depending on your starting fitness level. If you are new to exercise, listen to your own body and spend a few weeks/months gradually building up to this. Your body switches from using carbohydrates for energy to using stored fats for energy after about 20 minutes of aerobic activity, so if weight loss is your aim, building up duration is of importance. Some of these sessions can be a brisk walk into town or a vigorous housework session to your favourite music and doesn't always need to be structured activity. The main thing is to ensure that your heart and lungs are worked hard enough and long enough to gain the benefits of aerobic exercise, but not so long that you run the risk of injury. To check whether you are working out at the correct intensity try the talk test (see page 24);

you should be out of breath but still capable of speaking.

The following aerobic ball exercises can be performed in a couple of ways. You can either select some, and perform them individually in a circuit style for 30–60 seconds each, timing yourself with a stopwatch, or you can put them together into a choreographed routine. I have suggested a routine at the end of this chapter for you to try, but you could also have lots of fun putting together your own.

For either option, you need to choose a piece of music with a strong beat that will keep you working at a good brisk pace.

Before starting, ensure that you warm up by using some of the exercises in Chapter 1 (page 28–47) or by using some of the less vigorous exercises in this chapter at a gentle pace, gradually increasing intensity as your body warms up.

SEATED BOUNCES

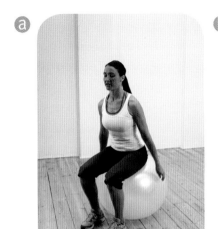 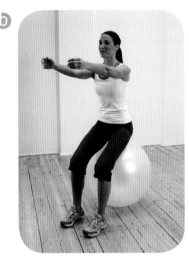

1 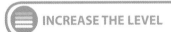 Start seated on your ball with your feet hip width apart and your arms relaxed by your sides.

2 Start a bouncing motion, swinging your arms to shoulder height and back in time with your bounces.

INCREASE THE LEVEL

1 Start off your bouncing motion as before, this time swing the arms higher and add a clap as they come up to head height.

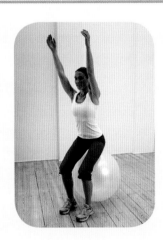

TIPS

- Try to get a rhythm going with your arms and your bouncing.
- Gradually make the bounces bigger, lifting your bottom slightly off the ball each time.

STEP TOUCH

1 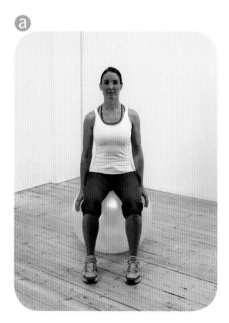 Start seated on the ball with your feet hip width apart and your hands lightly resting on the ball behind you.

2 Step your right foot out to the side, take the weight onto it, and then lightly tap your left foot in front.

3 Repeat on the other side, initiating a bouncing action as you move from side to side.

TIPS

- Use your hands to control and stabilise yourself on the ball.
- Start the movement gently and increase in vigour as your confidence grows.
- Keep your abdominal contraction in place to support the spine as you move from side to side.

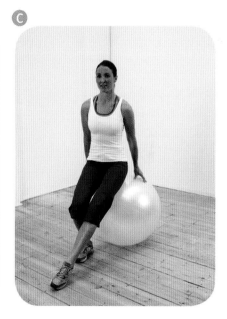
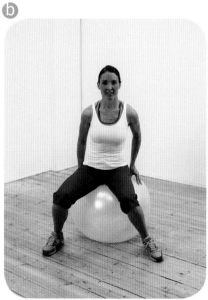

STAND UP SIT DOWNS

1 **ⓐ** Start seated on the ball with your feet hip width apart and your hands resting lightly on the ball behind you.

2 **ⓑ** Step your right foot out to the side taking the weight onto it. Lightly tap your left foot in front as you stand up, reaching your left arm up to the ceiling and keeping your right hand on the ball. **ⓒ**

3 Repeat on the other side, initiating a bouncing action as you move from side to side.

TIPS

- Keep your hand resting on the ball as you stand up to stop it from rolling away.
- You supporting leg will stay slightly bent as you stand up to enable you to keep contact with the ball.
- Keep your core contracted and ensure the spine stays neutral as you stand up.

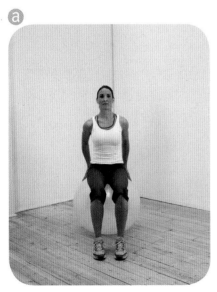
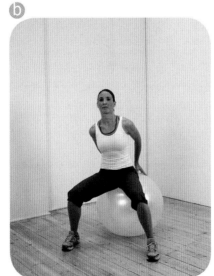
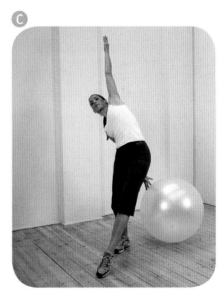

ROCKS FROM SIDE TO SIDE

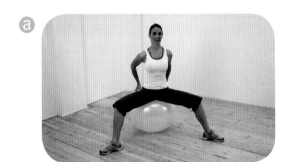

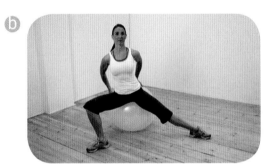

1 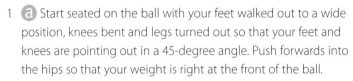 Start seated on the ball with your feet walked out to a wide position, knees bent and legs turned out so that your feet and knees are pointing out in a 45-degree angle. Push forwards into the hips so that your weight is right at the front of the ball.

2 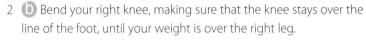 Bend your right knee, making sure that the knee stays over the line of the foot, until your weight is over the right leg.

3 Push into the floor activating the right thigh muscle, pushing yourself all the way over to the other side. You should now have your left knee bent and your right leg straight.

4 Continue pushing from side to side allowing the ball to roll underneath you.

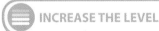 INCREASE THE LEVEL

1 Repeat steps 1 and 2 as before.
2 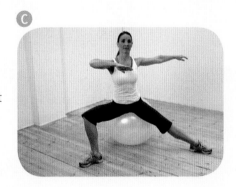 Now bring your arms up so that your right elbow is bent and your forearm is across your body and your left arm is extended out to the side.
3 As you change over to the left side, swap the arms so the left arm is bent and the right extended.
4 Repeat step 4 as before.

TIPS

- Keep your weight at the front of the ball throughout the exercise.
- Make sure that your knees stay over the line of your feet as they bend.
- If you want to make the exercises even harder you can try moving your arms overhead as you swap from side to side.

JACKS

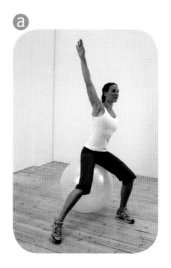
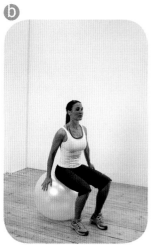

1 Start seated on your ball with your feet hip width apart and your arms relaxed by your sides.

2 Initiate a bouncing action. On the first bounce extend your right arm and right leg out sideways. On the second bounce bring them back to the starting position. **ⓑ**

3 Repeat on the left side and then continue from side to side in a steady rhythm.

INCREASE THE LEVEL

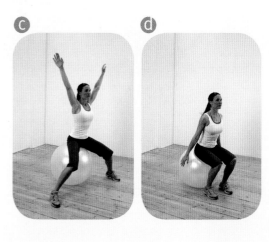

1 Repeat step 1 as before.
2 **ⓒ** Initiate a bouncing action again, this time on your first bounce jump both your legs out to the sides at the same time as extending your arms out to the sides.
3 **ⓓ** Now on your second jump, bring your feet back to their starting position at the same time as bringing your arms back in to your sides, ready to jump again.

TIPS

- Make sure your spine remains in neutral as you bounce.
- Keep your knees over the line of your toes as you jump out.
- Take gentle bounces at first, growing more vigorous as you gain confidence.

STANDING ARM LIFTS

1 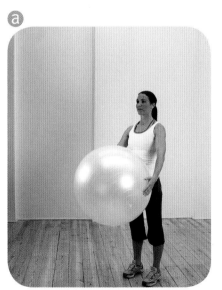 Start standing with your feet hip width apart and the ball held in front of you, with your arms relaxed down.

2 Raise your extended arms to chest height.

3 After a second's pause, raise them up so the ball is overhead.

4 Now lower them back to chest height.

5 Return to starting position.

TIPS

- Keep your torso still as the arms lift and lower. It is tempting to throw your weight back, but keeping your core contracted will ensure this doesn't happen.
- Keep the elbows slightly softened so you are not locking into the joint.
- Have a second's pause between each stage of the lifting and lowering. It should continue in a rhythmical motion in time with your music.

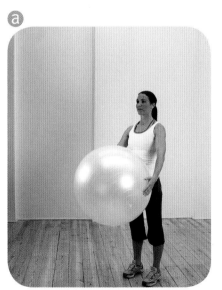

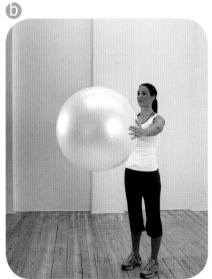

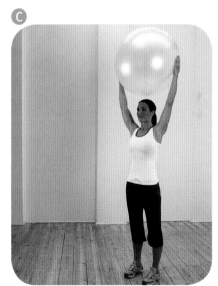

LUNGES WITH ARMS

1 **a** Start with your feet together, knees slightly bent and the ball held in front of your abdomen.

2 **b** Step your right foot back, keeping the front knee bent and at the same time punching the ball up overhead.

3 Step the right foot back in at the same time as bringing the ball back to your starting position.

4 Repeat on the left side and then continue alternating sides in a steady rhythm.

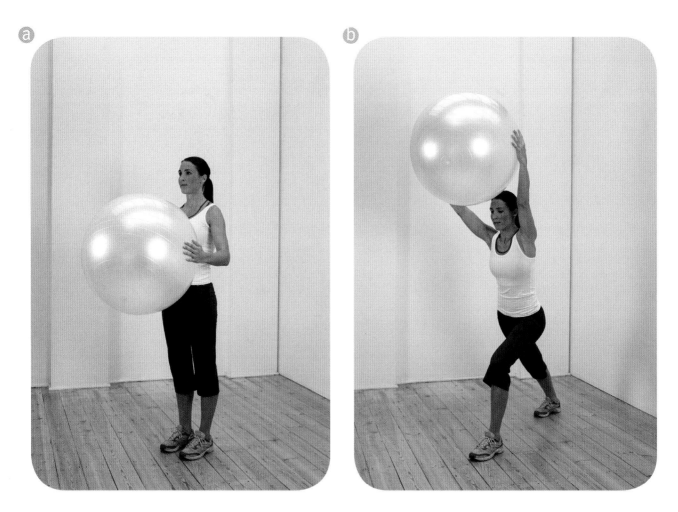

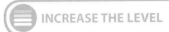
1   Repeat step 1 as before.
2   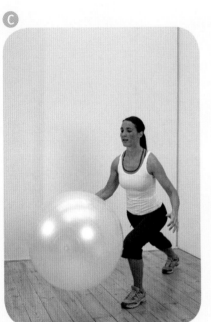c Step your right foot back into the lunge as before, this time bouncing the ball onto the floor at the same time.
3   d Bring the foot back in at the same time as catching the ball.
4   Repeat step 4 as before.

TIPS

- As you step your foot back, try and push the heel towards the floor, stretching up the back of the leg.
- Keep your core contraction in place; this will help control the movement, enabling you to go faster.

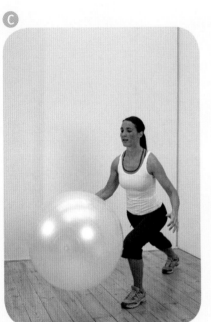

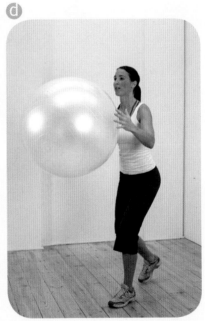

WALKS AROUND THE BALL

1 Start standing with the ball on the floor by your right foot and bend your knees so that you can lightly touch the ball with your right hand.

2 **b** **c** Take eight quick steps walking around the ball until you are back to the starting position.

3 Turn around and walk the other way around with your left hand on the ball.

4 Keep changing direction, taking eight steps to complete the circle.

TIP

- It is worth putting some music on for this one so that you have a beat to stay in time with!

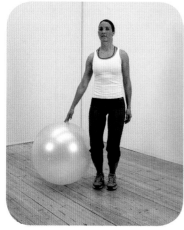

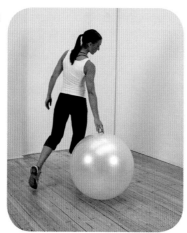

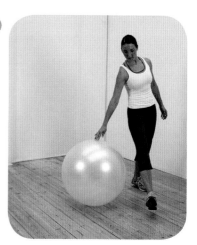

SWINGS SIDE TO SIDE

1 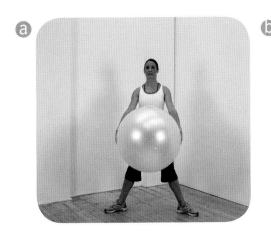 **a** Start standing with your feet wider than hip distance apart, legs slightly turned out. Hold the ball in front of you, arms relaxed down.

2 **b** Bend your knees and then swing the ball all the way up to the right side at the same time as transferring your weight onto your right leg and lightly tapping the left foot on the floor.

3 Swing the ball all the way down, bending your knees as you pass the centre **c**, then transferring your weight to your left leg and reaching the ball up to the left side. **d**

4 Keep swinging from side to side in a rhythmic motion.

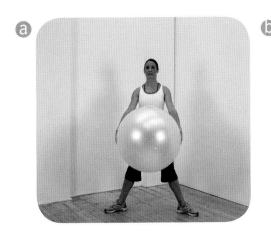

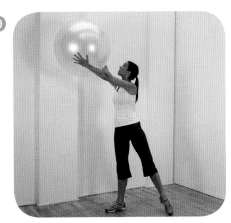

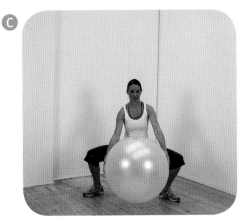

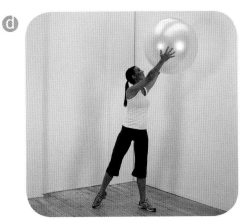

TIPS

- Make sure that your knees stay over the line of your feet when bent and passing centre.
- Don't bend your knees lower than a 90-degree angle.
- Keep your hips and shoulders square on to the front to avoid twisting of the spine.
- Try taking the swings half speed and double speed for variation.

SINGLE SIDE STEPS

1 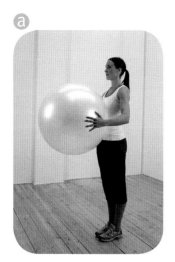 **a** Start standing with your feet together and the ball held at chest height close to your body.

2 **b** Step your right foot out to the side and at the same time push the ball forwards so your arms are now extended at chest height.

3 **c** Step your left foot in so the feet are together again and at the same time bring the arms back in to your chest.

4 Now repeat to the left and then continue alternating sides.

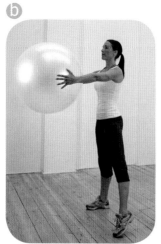

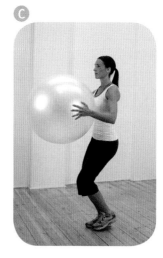

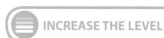 **INCREASE THE LEVEL**

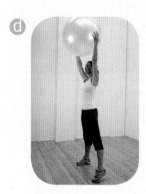

1 Repeat step 1 as before.
2 Step your right foot out to the side as before, but this time push the ball up overhead. **d**
3 As you close your left foot in, bring your arms back to the chest.
4 Repeat step 4 as before.

TIPS

- If you have trouble coordinating your arms and legs, try the legs alone to start with and then introduce the arms when you feel ready.
- You can try making up your own arm movements to add some fun!

DOUBLE SIDE STEPS

1 Start standing with your feet together and the ball held up above your head.

2 **b** Step your right foot out to the side at the same time as circling your arms down to the left.

3 **c** Now step your left foot in so the feet are together again and complete the circle with the arms bringing them back up above your head.

4 Repeat steps 2 and 3 again so that you have completed two steps to the right. Now take two side steps to the left, this time circling the arms down to the right and up the left side.

6 Continue the double side steps, alternating sides.

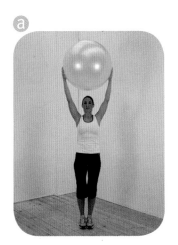
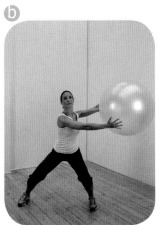
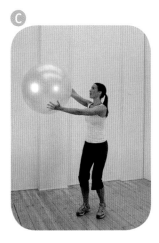

TIPS

- Get used to stepping with the feet alone before you introduce the arms.
- Keep the knees slightly relaxed as you step from side to side.
- Keep your hips and shoulders square on to the front as you move.

INCREASE THE LEVEL

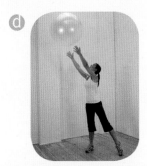

1 Repeat steps 1 to 3 as before.
2 **d** On your second side step, move the feet as before. The arms circle down to the left as before and then as they are circling back up, release and catch the ball as you are closing the feet.
3 Repeat to the left side.

MARCHING WITH BALL PUNCHES

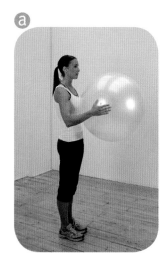

1 Start standing with your feet together and the ball in front of your chest.

2 ⓑ Start marching right, left, right, left and at the same time punch the ball forwards at chest height and then back in to your chest in time with your marching.

3 Keep marching to a steady rhythm or in time with your music.

INCREASE THE LEVEL

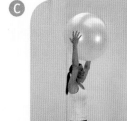

1 Repeat step 1 as before.
2 ⓒ Start marching as before, this time punch your arms up above your head and then back to chest height in time with your steps.
3 Repeat step 3 as before.

TIP

- If you struggle to coordinate your arms and legs, get used to one at a time and then join them together.

RUNNING AND BOUNCING

1 ⓐ Start standing with your feet together and your ball held in front of you.

2 ⓑ Run forwards for four steps starting with your right leg, at the same time bounce and catch your ball in time with your steps.

3 Now run backwards for four steps, still bouncing your ball.

4 Swap so that you start with your left leg after a few and try bouncing the ball with your other hand.

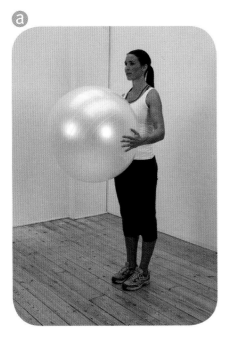

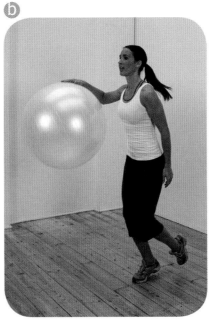

TIP

- Bounce the ball slightly to the side of your body so that you don't kick it with your foot when running.

GRAPEVINES

1 (a) Start standing with your feet together and the ball held in front of you.

2 (b) Step your right foot out to the side.

3 (c) Step your left foot behind your right.

4 (d) Step your right foot to the side again.

5 (e) Now step your left foot to join your right.

6 Repeat to the left and then alternate sides.

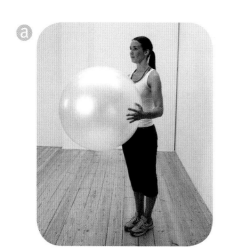

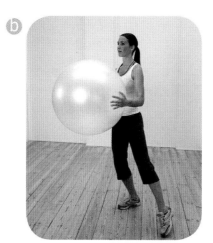

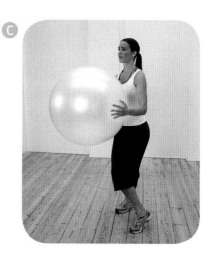

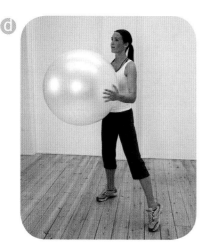

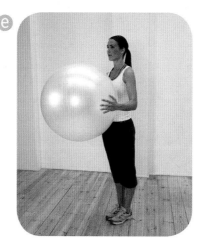

TIP

- This is all about coordination, so make sure you have mastered the legs before you add the arms.

1   Repeat step 1 as before.

2   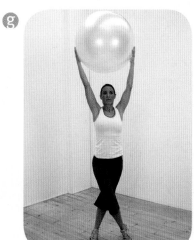 As you step your right foot out to the side, start to circle your arms to the right.

3   As your left foot steps behind, your arms should have continued the circle and be above your head.

4   As your right foot steps to the side again, your arms should have continued the circle and be halfway down on the left side.

5   As your left foot closes, your arms should have completed the circle.

6   Repeat on the left leg and circle the arms to the left.

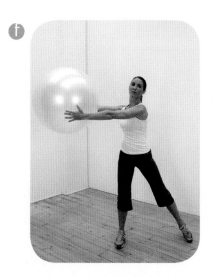
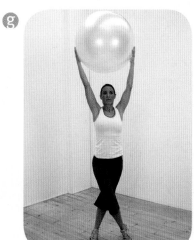
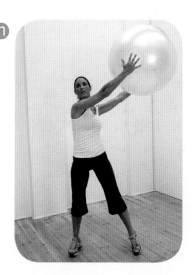

FOUR-STEP TURN

1 **a** Start standing with your feet together and the ball held out at chest height, arms extended.

2 **b** Step your right foot out to the side and turn a quarter turn to the right.

3 **c** Step your left foot joining the feet together and turning another quarter turn (you should be facing the back now).

4 **d** Step the right foot out again turning another quarter turn until you are facing the left side.

5 **e** Now step the left foot in again completing the turn.

6 Repeat starting with your left foot and turning to the left.

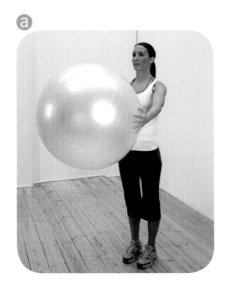

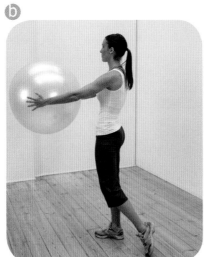

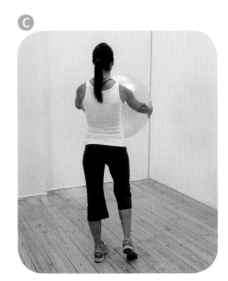

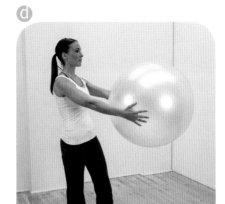

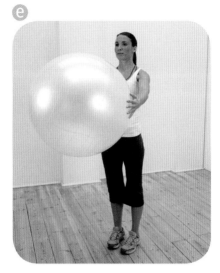

TIPS

- Try to make the turn one continuous movement.
- When the last foot steps in completing the turn, don't put all your weight onto it, as you want to immediately use it to start your turn in the opposite direction.

INCREASE THE LEVEL

1 Repeat step 1 as before.
2 Repeat all of the foot movements as before.
3 As you turn, allow the arms to circle up above your head **f** and then return to chest height by the end of each circle.

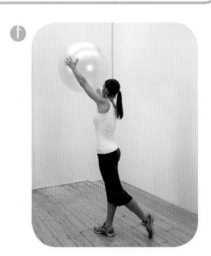

JUMP SQUATS

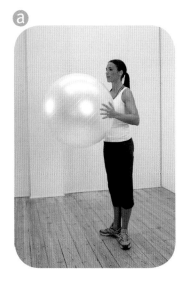

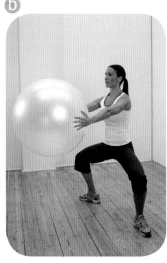

1 Start standing with your feet together in a turned out position and the ball held in front of you at chest height.

2 Jump your feet out wide and sit down into a squat, at the same time push the ball out in front of you at chest height, holding for three counts.

3 On the fourth count, jump your feet back to your starting position and bring the ball back in to your chest.

4 Repeat, jumping out on the first count and in on the fourth.

INCREASE THE LEVEL

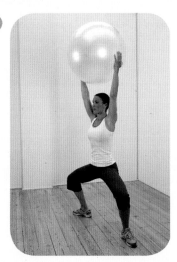

1 Repeat step 1 as before.
2 Repeat step 2 as before, but this time push the arms up so that the ball is overhead as you jump in the squat.
3 Repeat steps 3 and 4 as before.

TIPS

- When jumping into your squat, ensure that your knees stay over the line of your ankles and that you don't squat lower than a 90-degree angle at the knees.
- Keep the legs in a turned out position throughout the exercise.

HAMSTRING CURLS

1 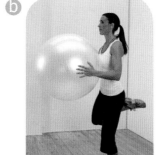 **(a)** Start standing with your knees bent, feet wider than hip width apart and the ball held in front of your chest.

2 **(b)** Move your weight over to your left leg, taking your right foot off the floor, bending your knee so that the heel of your right foot tries to touch your bottom while balancing on your left leg.

3 **(c)** Place your right foot back on the floor bending both knees again.

4 **(d)** Move your weight over to your right leg, taking the left foot off the floor and trying to touch your bottom.

5 Keep moving at a steady pace side to side.

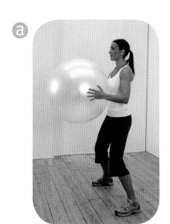 **(a)**

(b)

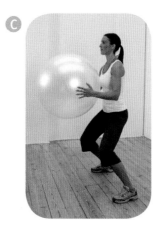 **(c)**

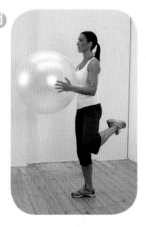 **(d)**

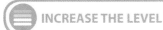 **INCREASE THE LEVEL**

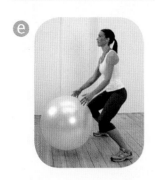 **(e)**

1 Repeat the exercise as before, but this time each time you bend both knees and pass the centre, bounce the ball and then catch it as you move onto one leg. **(e)**

TIP

- When you push onto one leg, keep the knee slightly relaxed so you do not jar the knee joint.

SALSA JUMPS

1 **ⓐ** Start standing with your feet hip width apart and the ball held in front of you with your arms relaxed down.

2 **ⓑ** Bend your knees and then jump to the right, curling your left leg behind you and bending the right knee slightly, keeping the leg forwards, landing on your right foot. At the same time as you jump, circle the ball up to the right side and overhead, coming down the left side and back to the starting position.

3 Place your left foot back to the starting position ready to jump again.

4 Repeat the jumps alternating sides.

TIP

- As you jump, try travelling sideways in the direction of the front leg to give a real salsa feel!

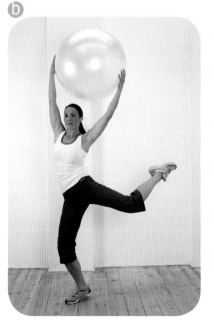

ⓐ ⓑ

DONKEY JUMPS WITH BALL BOUNCE

1 **ⓐ** Start standing with your feet hip width apart and the ball held in front of you with your arms relaxed down.

2 Lift your right foot off the floor behind you, **ⓑ** jump onto it and lift the left leg behind. **ⓒ** Place the left foot back on the floor ready to go again.

3 **ⓓ** Once you have got used to the jump, bounce the ball onto the floor in front of you as the first leg lifts each time, and then catch it as the second leg lifts.

4 Take a few jumps starting with the right leg, and then swap sides.

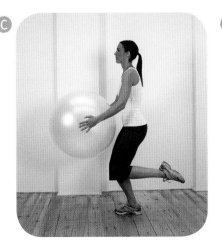

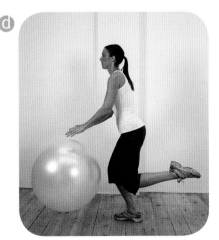

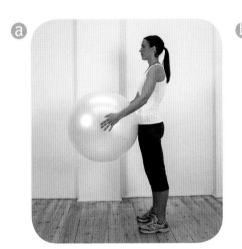

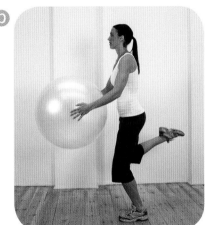

TIPS

- Imaging you are sweeping dirt off the floor with your feet as you swish them behind you.
- Get into a rhythm with the jumps; using music will again help here.

JUMPING KNEE LIFTS

1 Start standing with your feet hip width apart and the ball held in front of you with your arms relaxed down.

2 **ⓐ** Jump with both feet at the same time as lifting the ball up over your head. Jump again, this time landing on your left foot and bringing your right knee in towards your chest at the same time as bringing the arms back down. **ⓑ**

3 Jump again onto both feet bringing the ball up, and then this time on the second jump land on your right foot and lift your left knee.

4 Keep jumping in a steady rhythm alternating legs.

TIPS

- Use the force of moving the ball as momentum for lifting the knees.
- If you find this is too high impact on the knees, take the jumps out and make it more of a stepping motion.

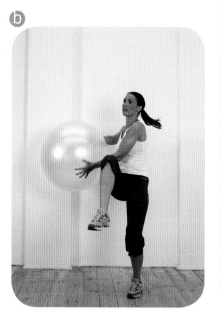

WALKING PLANK

1 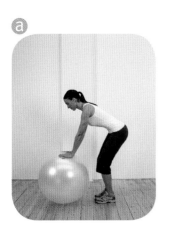 **a** Start standing with your hands placed on top of the ball and your knees slightly bent.

2 Walk your right leg out, **b** then your left so that you are in a press up position. **c**

3 Now walk your right leg back in **d** then your left. **e**

4 Pick up the ball and stand up with your arms up above your head. **f**

5 Now place the ball back to the floor, coming back to your starting position.

6 Repeat the whole exercise, keeping a steady rhythm.

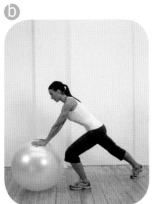

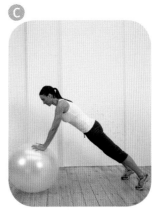

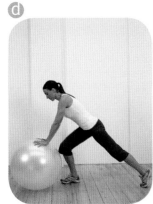

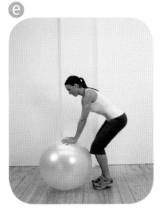

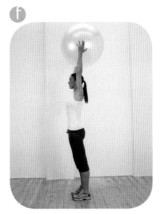

TIPS

- This exercise should be performed at a walking pace. Say to yourself right, left, right, left as the legs walk in and out to make sure you are keeping pace.
- When in the press up position, ensure your core contraction is in place to maintain neutral spine and avoid sagging in the middle.

COMPLETE ROUTINE

Now it is time to pick your favourite uplifting album, turn it on and have a go at linking some of the previous exercises together into a routine. It will take a few attempts to remember it all, but once you have learnt it you can repeat it as many times as you like.

The routine includes a seated section and a build up, where you repeat parts a few times before moving on to the next. It finishes with the final routine all the way through and this can be repeated as many times as you like.

I would also suggest you try adding some of your own choreography onto the end of it once you have it mastered. You can do this by either playing around with the exercises listed in the chapter or by making up some new ones!

 Seated bounces (page 98) x16

 Step touch (page 99) x8

 Seated bounces (page 98) x8

 Step touch (page 99) x8

 Seated bounces (page 98) x8

 Jacks (page 102) x8

 Seated bounces (page 98) x8

 Jacks (page 102) x8 – finish your last jack with your legs out wide

 Rocks from side to side (page 101) x16

 Step touch (page 99) x16 – finish with your feet hip width apart

 Stand up sit downs (page 100) x16 – finish standing up

 Walks around the ball (right) (page 106) x8 – pick the ball up on the eighth count

 Lunges with arms (page 104) x8

 Walks around the ball (left) (page 106) x8 – pick the ball up on the eighth count

 Lunges with arms (page 104) x8

Walk around the ball (right) (page 106) x8 – pick the ball up on the eighth count

 Lunges with arms (page 104) x8

 Walk around the ball (left) (page 106) x8 – pick the ball up on the eighth count

 Lunges with arms (page 104) x8

 Standing arm lifts (page 103) x8

 Swings side to side (page 107) x16

 Standing arm lifts (page 103) x8

 Swings side to side (page 107) x16

 Marching with ball punches (page 110) x16

 Running and bouncing (page 111) x2

 Marching with ball punches (page 110) x16

 Running and bouncing (page 111) x2

 Single side steps (page 108) x8

 Double side steps (page 109) x4

 Single side steps (page 108) x8

 Double side steps (page 109) x4

 Single side steps (page 108) x8

 Double side steps (page 109) x4

 Grapevines (page 112) x4

 Walking plank (page 121) x2

 Single side steps (page 108) x8

 Double side steps (page 109) x4

 Grapevines (page 112) x4

 Walking plank (page 121) x2

 Single side steps (page 108) x4

 Four-step turn (page 114), 1 x right 1 x left

 Hamstring curls (page 117) x8

 Single side steps (page 108) x4

 Four-step turn (page 114), 1 x right 1 x left

 Hamstring curls (page 117) x8

Single side steps (page 108) x4

Four-step turn (page 114), 1 x right 1 x left

Hamstring curls (page 117) x8

Single side steps (page 108) x4

Four-step turn (page 114), 1 x right 1 x left

Hamstring curls (page 117) x8

Double side steps (page 109) x2

Jump squats (page 116) x2

Salsa jumps (page 118) x4

Double side steps (page 109) x2

Jump squats (page 116) x2

Salsa jumps (page 118) x4

Double side steps (page 109) x2

Jump squats (page 116) x2

Double side steps (page 109) x2

Jump squats (page 116) x2

Salsa jumps (page 118) x4

Grapevines (page 112) x2

Jumping knee lifts (page 120) x4

Grapevines (page 112) x2

Donkey jumps with ball bounce (page 119) x4

Grapevines (page 112) x2

Jumping knee lifts (page 120) x4

Grapevine (page 112) x2

Donkey jumps with ball bounce (page 119) x4

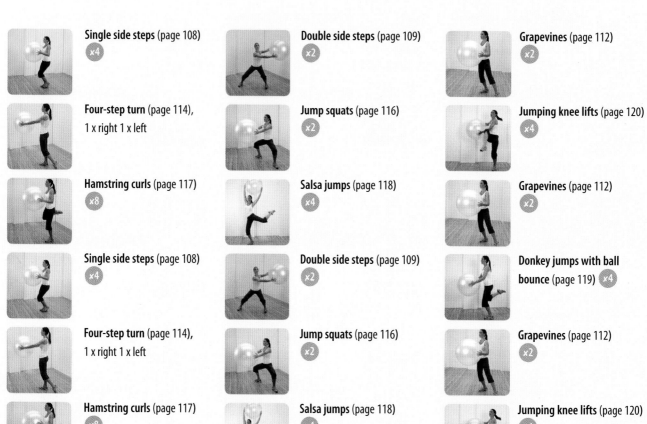

Single side steps (page 108)

 Double side steps (page 109)

 Double side steps (page 109)

Jump squats (page 116)

 Grapevines (page 112)

Salsa jumps (page 118)

 Walking plank (page 121)

Grapevines (page 112)

 Single side steps (page 108)

Jumping knee lifts (page 120)

 Four-step turn (page 114),
1 x right, 1 x left

Grapevines (page 112)

 Hamstring curls (page 117)

**Donkey jumps with ball
bounce** (page 119)

CHAPTER FOUR

PILATES WITH THE BALL

WHAT IS PILATES?

Pilates is a complete and thorough programme of mental and physical conditioning. It offers a different way of thinking about your body and, through practising the movements, you will gain a better understanding of your personal strengths and weaknesses.

What makes the Pilates method so attractive is that it is versatile and speaks to all ages and abilities. Programmes can be designed to help people recovering from injuries or can be intensely challenging for seasoned athletes. Its accessibility, however, means that the kind of people who come to Pilates wouldn't normally step foot in a gym or fitness class.

PILATES ON THE BALL

There is nothing forced or unnatural about adapting Pilates to the exercise ball. They both have links to physiotherapy and are both primarily concerned with aligning the body and training our deep postural muscles.

The Pilates method has both mat-based and machine-based routines, although most people who have come across Pilates would probably have taken part in a matwork-based class. The machine-based or 'reformer' Pilates is less well known and happens on very specialised equipment found only in dedicated Pilates or dance studios.

What is great about combining Pilates with the ball is that you can easily recreate some of the 'reformer' Pilates

exercises on the round surface of the ball, as well as adding an extra dimension to the matwork exercises. Pilates on the ball will create a long, lean body shape by continuously lengthening through the body to stay balanced and poised.

Pilates, just like the ball, is distinctive in as much as it will systematically train all the muscle groups in the body. It will train the weak muscles as well as the strong, the small as well as the large. Think back to if you or someone you know has ever spent hours in the gym training hard without injury, but then come home and picked up something relatively light, only to pull a muscle. This is because traditional exercises do not prepare our bodies for the kind of activity required for 'functional movement' (see page 8). Instead we train our body as separate parts, one muscle at a time, but we don't train our body to work in synergy.

Both Pilates and the ball train our bodies in 'functional movement' rather than in movements that we will never use in our everyday life. Through self-awareness we can identify our bad habits, maintain a healthy body and create natural poise.

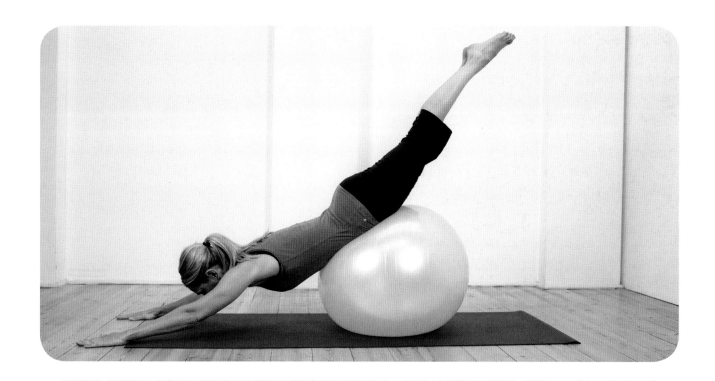

WHO WAS JOSEPH PILATES?

Joseph Pilates was born in Mönchengladbach, Germany in 1883. He was a sickly child who suffered from a number of debilitating conditions including rickets, asthma and rheumatic fever. He was determined not to allow poor health to cloud his future, so was devoted to becoming as fit and strong as humanly possible.

In 1912 Joseph Pilates moved to England where he worked initially as a boxer, then a circus performer, followed by a self-defence trainer for detectives. During World War 1 he was held in an internment camp, but became a nurse and trained other interns in physical fitness. His physical training of these inmates was apparently widely credited as the reason none of them succumbed to the 1918 influenza pandemic that killed thousands. He improvised, making exercise equipment out of bedsprings, attaching them to the walls above the bed so that patients could exercise while lying down.

After the war, Pilates continued his work back in Germany before moving to America in 1926. On the ship to New York he met his future wife, Clara, a nurse.

Joseph Pilates set up an exercise studio on Eighth Avenue and by the 1940s had made a name for himself within the dance community, counting many of New York's finest dancers among his clients.

He died in 1967 at the age of 83. Clara carried on what was already known as the Pilates Studio in New York and in the 1970s Romana Kryzanowska, a former student, became the director.

THE EIGHT PRINCIPLES OF PILATES

These eight principles are the cornerstone of the Pilates method. Bear these in mind when executing each exercise, and it is likely that you will adopt the correct techniques and gain maximum results. Quotes are from Joseph Pilates.

1. Concentration

'Always keep your mind wholly concentrated on the purpose of the exercises as you perform them.'

Pilates is the thinking way of moving and therefore requires a different kind of concentration than other fitness styles. The benefits of improving your concentration are well worth the effort. It will reduce stress levels and you will have better clarity of thought and mental focus.

2. Breathing

'Breathing is the first act of life. Our very life depends on it. Millions have never learnt to master the art of correct breathing.'

Pilates will teach you new breathing techniques. We need to keep our core contracted while performing Pilates, as this is how we strengthen and protect the spine. With the core contracted we can no longer direct our breath into the abdominal area so we instead direct it into the ribcage. This is called thoracic breathing (see page 24).

3. Centring

'Pilates develops the body uniformly, corrects wrong postures, restores physical vitality, invigorates the mind and elevates the spirit.'

Joseph Pilates believed that our abdominal muscles were the powerhouse of our body. They are our centre and therefore every movement is initiated from them. To maintain a strong centre you must have equal strength between your abdominals and your back.

4. Control

'Good posture can be successfully acquired only when the entire mechanism of the body is under perfect control.'

Control is learnt right from when we take our first shaky steps as a child. With control we can start to take charge of our bodies. Unfortunately over time we pick up bad habits, but through Pilates we can take a step back and re-learn.

5. Precision

'The benefits of Pilates depend solely on your performing the exercises exactly according to the instructions.'

Pilates movements are exact, and demand precise actions and breathing. Think of synchronised swimmers or of the exact choreography that dancers learn. Through Pilates you will gain an appreciation of precision skills and an awareness of space and timing.

6. Movement

'Designed to give you suppleness, grace and skill that will be unmistakably reflected in the way you walk, the way you play and in the way you work.'

Pilates is slow, graceful and controlled. The movements should be continuous, having no beginning or end. Imagine a wheel turning round and round; you cannot tell where the movement starts or where it ends. Nothing should be sharp, strained or forced.

7. Isolation

'Each muscle may cooperatively and loyally aid in the uniform development of all our muscles.'

When we talk about isolation in Pilates we are just making sure that we identify all our muscles for ourselves. Pilates exercises ensure that we develop the weaker areas of the body alongside opposing, stronger muscles.

8. Routine

'Make up your mind that you will perform your Pilates movements 10 minutes each day without fail.'

Pilates works best when complementing your current exercise programme. It does however only work if you practise and make it a regular part of your routine.

BREATHING PRACTICE

In Pilates we attempt to slow down the breath, increase the depth of respiration and coordinate breathing with our movements.

We also focus on our core contraction and neutral spine alignment as we do with our work on the ball (see pages 16–19). It is because of this contraction in the abdominals that we need to direct our breathing into the ribcage.

Please refer back to pages 24–27 for the breathing exercises. It would be beneficial for you to refresh yourself with these exercises before starting any Pilates work on the ball.

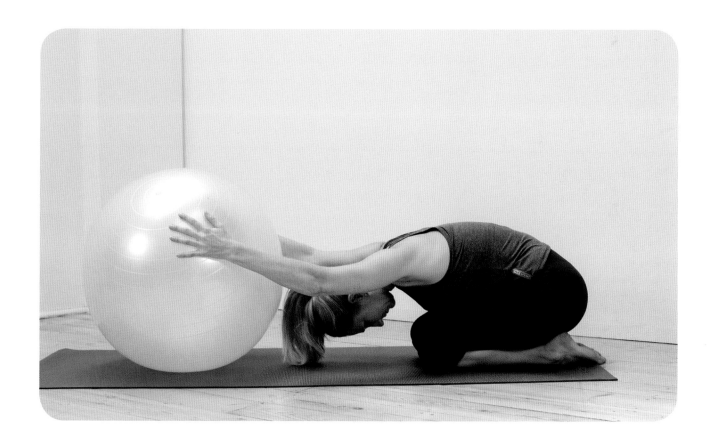

TO START

The following exercises are great to use as a warm up and to focus the mind and body. They are also a good place to start if you have not taken part in any Pilates-based exercises before, and can be used to master your neutral spine position, core contraction and coordination of breath and movement before moving on to more challenging exercises.

PELVIC TILTS

? **WHAT FOR?** To mobilise the pelvis and practise moving in and out of a neutral spine posture.

1 **a** Start seated on the ball in neutral position with your knees bent and feet hip width apart.

2 **b** Breathe in to prepare, then breathe out as you slowly tilt your pelvis forwards, allowing the ball to roll under you.

3 Breathe in as you return the pelvis to neutral.

4 **c** Now breathe out again as you tilt the pelvis back, allowing the ball to roll with you.

5 Breathe in again as you return to the centre.

6 Repeat the tilts 4–6 times.

TIPS

- Make sure you are sitting tall on your sitting bones before you start (these are the bony bits that you can feel underneath your bottom when sitting on a hard floor).
- Imagine you are lengthening through the crown of the head, and that you grow a little taller each time you return to centre.
- Keep your core contraction in place throughout, it will help you find your neutral position more easily.

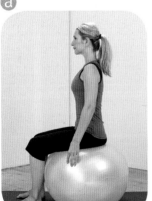
a

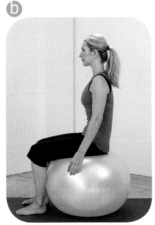
b

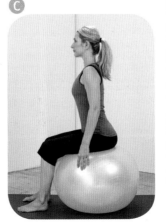
c

SPINE TWIST

? WHAT FOR? To mobilise the spine, a great exercise to concentrate on isolating the upper body while the hips stay rooted on the ball.

1 Start seated tall on the ball with your knees bent, feet hip width apart and your arms bent in front of you, opposite hand touching opposite elbow.

2 Breathe in to prepare, then breathe out as you turn your upper body to the right side as far as you can without allowing the hips to move.

3 Breathe in again when you reach your furthest point of the twist, then breathe out again as you turn back to your starting position.

4 Repeat the exercise 4–6 times, alternating sides.

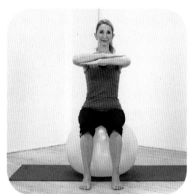

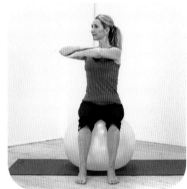

 INCREASE THE LEVEL

1 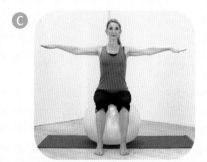 Start seated on your ball as in step 1, but this time have your arms lengthened out to the side at shoulder height.
2 Repeat steps 2–4 as before.

TIPS

- Make sure your hips and knees stay square on to the front throughout the exercise.
- Try to think about growing taller through the crown of the head each time you return to centre.
- Keep your nose line level throughout. Visualise that you have chalk on the end of your nose and are drawing a level horizontal line around the wall as you twist.
- Keep the spine lengthened throughout, don't allow the body to sink down as you grow tired.

KNEE LIFTS WITH BALL ROLL

? **WHAT FOR?** To mobilise the knee joints and to test your centre of gravity and balancing skills on the ball.

1 **a** Start sitting on the ball with your knees bent and your feet hip width apart. Have your hands resting lightly on the sides of the ball. Lift your right foot a few inches off the floor.

2 **b** Breathe in as you push back on your supporting leg, extending it as far as possible.

3 **c** Breathe out again as you roll the ball back in by pushing the supporting heel into the floor.

4 Repeat the rolls out and in 6–8 times and then repeat on the other leg.

TIPS

- To stay balanced on the ball you will need to lengthen long through the body – imagine a string through the crown of your head pulling you towards the ceiling. You will also need to keep your core contracted to stabilise the torso, stopping you from wobbling.
- If you find this difficult, keep the movement small until you have built up a bit more confidence.

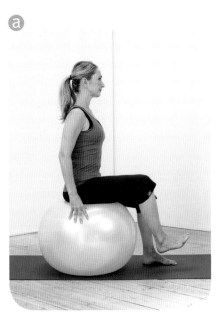

a

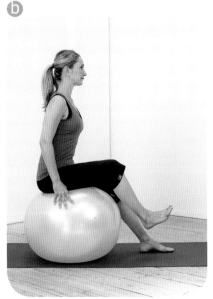

b

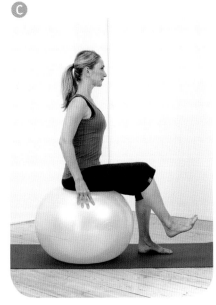

c

SIDE BEND

? **WHAT FOR?** To mobilise and stretch though the spine and lengthen down the sides of the body.

1 **a** Start seated on the ball with your knees bent and your feet hip width apart. Breathe in as you reach your right arm up above your head.

2 **b** Breathe out as you bend to the left as far as is comfortable. Breathe in again, holding this position.

3 Breathe out as you return to your starting position. Repeat the side bend 4–6 times, alternating sides.

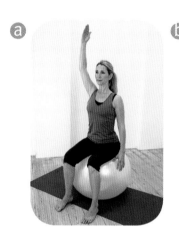

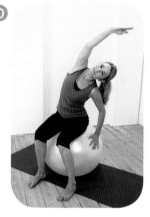

TIPS

- Think about lengthening long through the finger as you bend to the side so that you are keeping an elongation through the spine.
- As you bend, push the opposite hip into the ball so it does not lift off. Keep the hips and knees square on to the front throughout.
- As you return to your starting position think about initiating the movement from the abdominals or your core contraction.

INCREASE THE LEVEL

1 Repeat steps 1 and 2 as before.
2 **c** As you breathe out, drop your chest towards the floor, feeling a stretch in the upper back.
3 Breathe in as you come back to your side bend position.
4 **d** Then breathe out again as you lift your chest, looking up to the ceiling.
5. Breathe in as you return to your side bend position again.
6. Breathe out as you return to your starting position.
7. Repeat 4–6 times alternating sides.

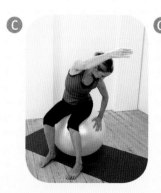

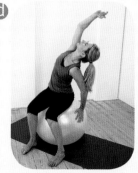

THE SAW

> **? WHAT FOR?** To mobilise and stretch through the spine and to stretch up the backs of the legs. A great exercise for improving posture.

1 **a** Start seated on the ball with your knees bent, feet hip width apart and your arms out to the sides at shoulder height.

2 **b** Breathe in as you rotate the upper body to the right in a spine twist.

3 **c** Breathe out as you extend your right leg and tilt the torso forwards so that you are reaching towards your right foot with your left hand.

4 **d** Breathe in again as you return to your spine twist position, placing your right foot back on the floor.

5 Breathe out as you return to your starting position.

6 Repeat the saw 4–6 times, alternating sides.

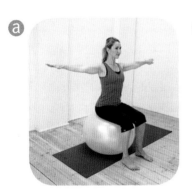
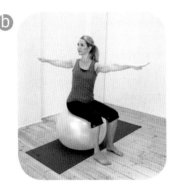
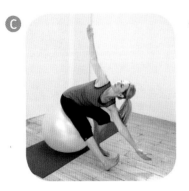
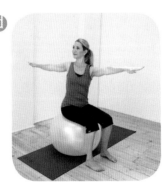

TIPS

- Make sure that your sitting bones are firmly on the ball when you start and try not to let the ball drift from this position during the movement.
- When reaching towards your foot, make sure the arm position is the same as in the spine twist. You should just tilt the whole shape forwards in one piece.
- Think about growing taller each time you return to the centre.

ARM CIRCLES

 WHAT FOR? To mobilise the shoulders and to challenge neutral spine position.

1 Start sitting on your ball with your feet hip width apart. Walk yourself forwards on the ball allowing it to roll up your spine until it is resting underneath the back of your neck. Make sure that your hips are lifted in a straight line with your shoulders and knees. Once in position, lift your arms up so they are reaching towards the ceiling. **a**

2 Breathe in as you lengthen your arms above your head. **b**

3 Then breathe out as you continue the circle all the way around until you are back to your starting position.

4 Repeat the circles 6–8 times.

TIPS

- Keep your core contraction in place to maintain the neutral position of the spine. As the arms circle back it is very easy to allow the back to arch, so concentration will be needed here!
- Keep your hips lifted throughout the exercise so that they remain level with your knees and shoulders.

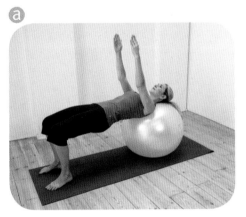

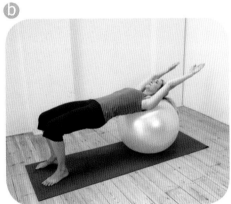

SHOULDER ISOLATIONS

? WHAT FOR? To work on isolating the shoulders, allowing them to push down the back. A great exercise if you are someone who suffers from tension in this area.

1 Start sitting on your ball with your feet hip width apart. Walk yourself forwards on the ball, allowing it to roll up your spine until it is resting underneath the back of your neck. Make sure that your hips are lifted in a straight line with your shoulders and knees. Once in position, lift your arms up so they are reaching towards the ceiling. **a**

2 Squeeze your shoulder blades together, hold for a couple of seconds. **b**

3 Now release the position, coming back to neutral.

4 Keep squeezing and releasing for 8–10 repetitions, then walk yourself back up off the ball.

TIPS

- This is a very subtle movement, just try and practise isolating the shoulders while everything else stays held in place.
- You can really use the ball here as something to push against as you squeeze.
- Also concentrate on keeping your neutral spine position throughout.

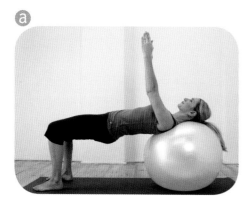

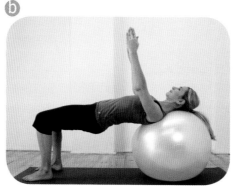

HIP ROTATIONS

? **WHAT FOR?** To mobilise the hips and increase flexibility in the inner thigh muscles.

1 **a** Start lying on your back with your arms relaxed by your sides and your knees bent, feet placed onto the ball. Once in position allow your knees to open out to the sides as far as you feel comfortable.

2 **b** Breathe in as you push the ball away extending the legs in a turned out position.

3 **c** Now breathe out as you rotate from the hips so the legs are in a turned in position, and then pull the ball back in.

4 Allow the knees to fall back out to your starting position.

5 Repeat the rotations 6–8 times.

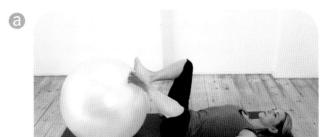

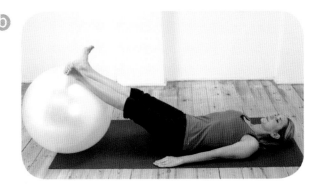

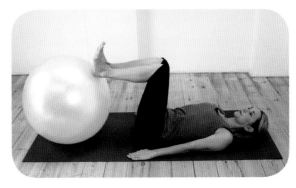

TIPS

- Keep your spine in neutral to avoid any overarching of the back while extending the legs.
- Take the exercise slowly, really finding the opportunity to mobilise the hips at your own pace.

SPINE CURLS

1 **(a)** Start lying on your back with your arms relaxed by your sides and your feet placed onto the ball.

2 **(b)** Breathe in to prepare, then breathe out as you lift the hips off the floor, rolling up through the spine until you are in a straight diagonal line from your shoulders to your knees.

3 Breathe in at the top, then breathe out again as you roll back down through the spine one vertebra at a time, returning to your starting position.

4 Repeat the spine curls 6–8 times.

TIPS

- Keep the movement steady and controlled, trying to maintain the same pace throughout.
- Concentrate on feeling each vertebra as you unpeel and then replace the spine onto the floor. Work on any areas of the spine that feel stiff.
- Get a good base of support on the ball by having your feet hip width apart or wider if necessary.

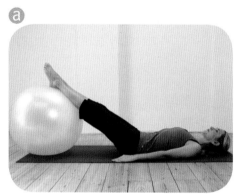

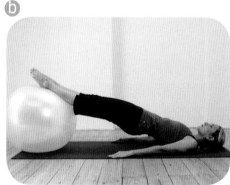

MOVING ON

The following exercises will provide more of a challenge and should be introduced gradually into your routine at your own pace. Some exercises you will initially find challenging, if not impossible, but allow your body time to build up strength and core stability and you will be surprised at how quickly you progress.

THE HUNDRED

? **WHAT FOR?** To strengthen the core muscles, giving definition to the abdominals.

1 **a** Start seated on the ball with your knees bent and your feet hip width apart. Walk yourself out on the ball, allowing it to roll up your spine, stopping when the ball is resting underneath your upper back.

2 **b** Breathe in to prepare and as you breathe out, curl the upper body up, reaching your arms towards the opposite wall, palms facing down.

3 **c** Now holding the position, make a small beating movement with the arms, moving them up and down by a few inches in a rhythmic motion. Breathe in for five beats, then out for five.

4 Keep beating the arms until you get to a hundred beats (you can build up gradually to this amount).

TIPS

- Try to keep the torso still as the arms move.
- Don't let the ball bounce around underneath you, this would be a sign that you have lost control of the movement.
- If you feel there is too much strain on your neck in this position, try taking one hand behind your head to support it and taking the beats with one arm, swapping arms when you reach 50.

a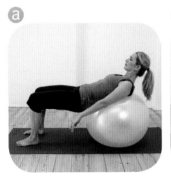

b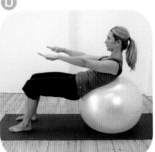

c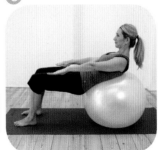

BACK ROWING

? WHAT FOR? To mobilise the spine and strengthen the core muscles.

1 **ⓐ** Start seated on the ball with your knees bent and your feet hip width apart. Lengthen your arms out to the sides to start.

2 **ⓑ** Breathe in to prepare, then as you breathe out, round the spine and curl back on the ball, bringing the arms together in the centre.

3 **ⓒ** Breathe in here, then breathe out as you come all the way up, past centre and over the knees, keeping the spine rounded throughout the movement.

4 Breathe in again as you come back up to the centre, extending the spine again and opening the arms back out into your starting position.

5 Repeat the rowing 6–8 times.

ⓐ
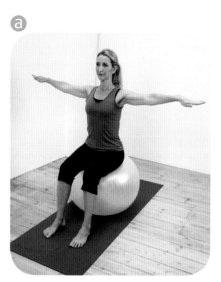

ⓑ
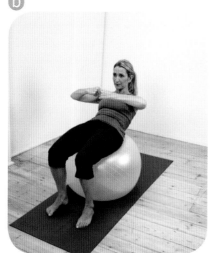

ⓒ
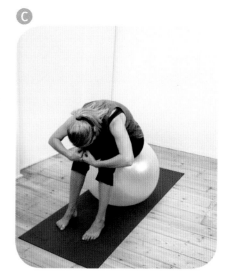

INCREASE THE LEVEL

1 Repeat steps 1 and 2 as before.
2 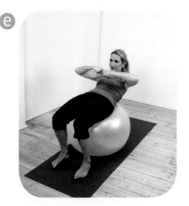 Inhale in this position, this time as you exhale, twist to the right side as you lift up to a 45-degree angle and reach out with the arms.
3 Breathe in and come back to the centre.
4 Breathe out and twist to the left, this time lifting to 45-degrees and reaching with the arms.
5 Breathe in and come to centre again.
6 Breathe out as you curl all the way up, past centre and over the knees, keeping the spine rounded throughout the movement.
7 Repeat steps 4 and 5 as before.

TIPS

- Try to keep the ball stabilised throughout, so that it is rolling only as much as necessary to execute the exercise.
- Try to initiate the lifting and twisting movements from your abdominals, avoiding the temptation to jerk the arms and upper body to help you lift up more easily.
- Keep the neck in line with the spine and try to avoid too much tension in this area.

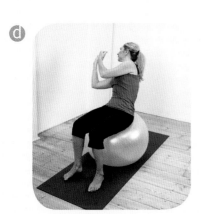

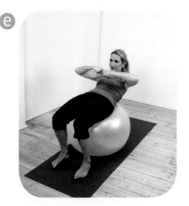

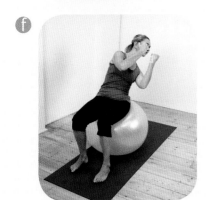

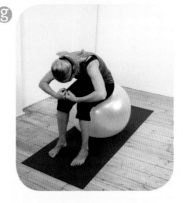

THE HEDGEHOG

? WHAT FOR? This exercise is a real test of all over body strength, balance and control.

1   Start on your hands and knees over the ball.

2 Walk out onto your hands so that the ball rolls down your legs until the ball is underneath your thighs. Make sure your hands are directly under your shoulders.

3 Breathe in to prepare, then breathe out as you bend your knees and roll the ball in towards your hands, lifting your hips up towards the ceiling.

4 Breathe in again as you roll the ball back out, keeping the abdominal contracted and neutral spine position.

5 Repeat the rolls 6–8 times.

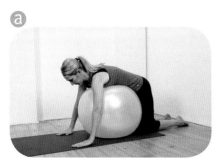

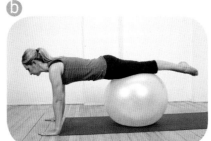

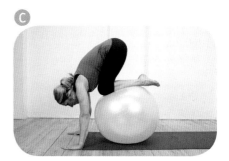

INCREASE THE LEVEL

1 Repeat steps 1 and 2 as before.
2 Breathe in to prepare, and this time as you roll the ball in, keep the legs straight so you are coming into a pike position, sending your hips up to the ceiling.
3 Repeat steps 4 and 5 as before.

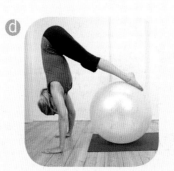

TIPS

- Initiate the rolling in of the ball by contracting your abdominals and draw in the legs using the core muscles.
- Keep the exercise controlled throughout, and keep a constant speed.
- When returning to your start position after each roll, ensure you are not arching into the lower back.

THE SWAN DIVE

 WHAT FOR? This exercise uses the whole body as an integrated unit and demands upper body and core strength as well as total body control. It is a lovely exercise which integrates the whole body into one movement. When you get it right it actually feels quite liberating!

1 **a** Start on your hands and knees over the ball.

2 **b** Walk out onto your hands so that the ball rolls down your legs until the ball is underneath your thighs. Rotate your legs from your hips so that they are slightly turned out.

3 **c** Breathe in and lift your chest slightly towards the ceiling.

4 **d** Now breathe out and push back on your hands, drawing your legs up behind you to form a straight diagonal line from hands to feet.

5 Breathe in again as you return to your starting position.

6 Repeat 6–8 times.

TIPS

- Try to keep your head in line with the rest of your spine throughout the exercise.
- Use the heel of your hands to initiate the movements of rolling out and in.
- Try to feel an extension throughout the whole body when in the swan dive position.
- In your fully extended position maintain your neutral spine.

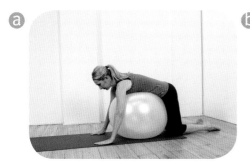

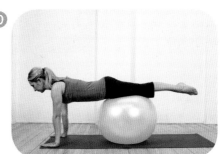

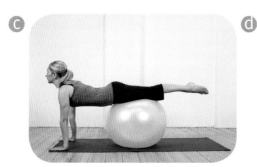

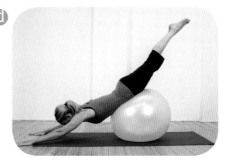

KNEELING OPPOSITE ARM AND LEG EXTENSIONS

? WHAT FOR? To practise centring the weight and integrating the whole body into a movement.

1 **a** Start on your hands and knees over the ball.

2 **b** Breathe in to prepare, then breathe out as you lengthen your right arm and left leg along the floor until they are both fully extended.

3 Breathe in as you slide the arm and leg back in to your starting position.

4 Repeat the exercise 6–8 times alternating sides.

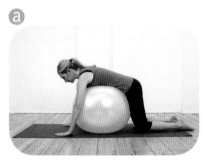

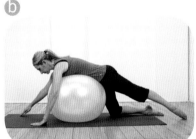

TIP

- The idea of this exercise is to keep your weight even through your hands and knees. When you remove your opposite hand and knee from the floor your weight should stay exactly where it is and should not shift over your supporting knee. This is achieved by holding tight in the centre and fully lengthening the arm and leg away from you, rather than thinking of a lifting movement. Use a mirror to check there is no side-to-side movement to ensure this is happening.

≡ INCREASE THE LEVEL

1 Repeat step 1 as before.
2 **c** Repeat step 2, but this time keep extending away until your right foot and left hand come away from the floor and lift until they are shoulder/hip height.
3 Repeat steps 3 and 4 as before.

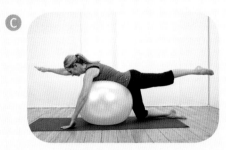

BALL BALANCE

1 Start lying on your back and try to place the ball so that it is resting on the soles of your feet.

2 Ⓑ Now try and extend your legs keeping balance of the ball, resting your arms on the floor.

3 Stay balanced here as long as you feel comfortable!

TIPS

- Adjust your feet when you first place them on the ball so that they are slightly turned out and a few inches apart at the heels. This will give you a good base of support on which to balance the ball.
- Try to keep your breathing steady and even while balancing.

Ⓐ
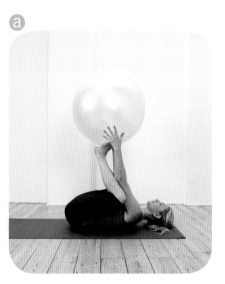

Ⓑ
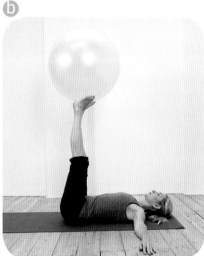

FOOTWORK

> **? WHAT FOR?** To tone and strengthen the legs, bottom and abdominal muscles. Great for long lean legs!

1 **a** Start lying on your back, with your arms relaxed by your sides and your feet resting on the ball with your knees bent.

2 **b** Breathe in to prepare, then as you breathe out, slowly roll the ball away from you, extending the legs and flexing the feet.

3 **c** Breathe in again as you roll the ball back in.

4 Repeat the rolls 6–8 times.

5 **d** Now go back to your starting position and turn the legs out so your heels are touching, but your hips, knees and feet are rotated out to a 45-degree angle.

6 **e** Repeat steps 2 and 3 as before, keeping the legs turned out. Then repeat the turned out rolls 6–8 times.

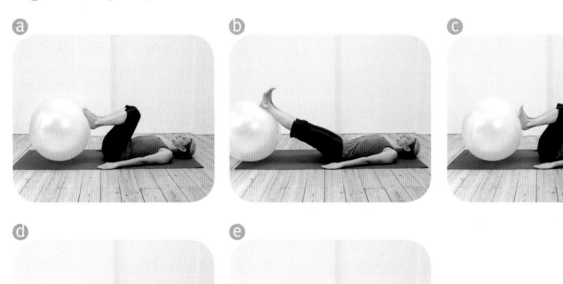

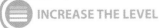
1 Repeat step 1 as before, first in the turned in position.
2 **f** Breathe in to prepare, then as you breathe out, slowly roll the ball away from you, extending the legs and flexing the feet and lifting the hips off the floor until you are in a straight diagonal line from shoulders to feet.
3 Repeat steps 3 and 4 as before.
4 **g** Repeat in the turned out position.

TIPS

- Keep your core engaged so your spine stays neutral throughout. Check that your lower back is not arching away from the floor by placing your hand by the small of your back and making sure there is only a very small gap (enough for a piece of paper to slip through).
- Think of lengthening the legs away from you, imaging you are being pulled in opposite directions from head to toe so that a lengthening happens right through the body.
- When lifting the hips away from the floor, remember to roll slowly up and down through the spine working through each and every vertebra.

f

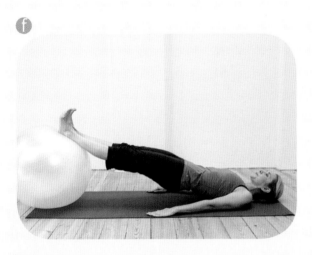

g

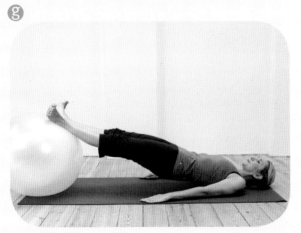

ONE LEG CIRCLE

? WHAT FOR? To tone and strengthen the muscles in the legs and to challenge overall body control and stability.

1 **(a)** Start by lying on the floor with the ball underneath your lower legs and your arms relaxed by your sides.

2 **(b)** Breathe in as you place your right foot on your left knee.

3 **(c)** Then breathe out as you extend your right leg out to a 45-degree angle.

4 **(d)** Now take small circles outwards with the leg, breathing in as you take the first half of the circle and out on the second half.

5 Take 6–8 circles in this direction, then reverse the direction of the leg and take 6–8 more.

6 To come out of the position, bring the right foot back to the left knee and place the foot back onto the ball.

7 Repeat the exercise on the other leg.

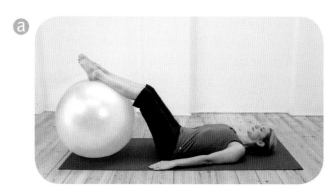

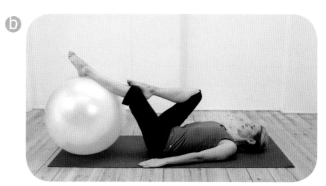

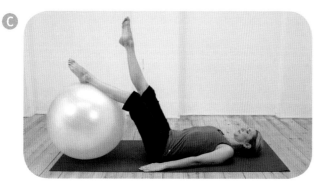

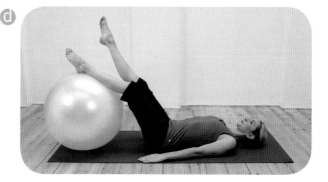

1 Repeat step 1 as before.
2 **e** Breathe in to prepare and then breathe out as you roll up through the spine, lifting the hips off the floor until your body is in a straight diagonal line from shoulders to toes.
3 **f** Repeat steps 2 and 3 as before, keeping the hips lifted.
4 Repeat steps 4–7 as before.

f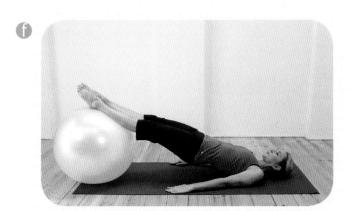

g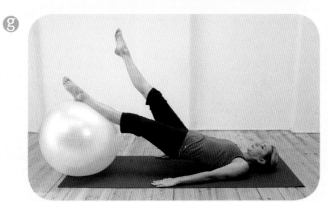

TIPS

- Try to keep the circles small, controlled and at a constant speed throughout.
- Keep your arms and hands relaxed and avoid the temptation to push against the floor.
- When taking the more difficult level, ensure your spine is supported by your core contraction throughout and the body is stabilised with only the non-supporting leg moving.

SHORT SPINE PREPARATION

? WHAT FOR? To strengthen and tone the lower abdominal muscles and the legs. This exercise will also really challenge your neutral spine position.

1 Start lying on your back with your arms relaxed by your sides. Hold the ball between your lower legs and bend the knees, lifting the ball off the floor.

2 Breathe in to prepare, then breathe out as you extend the legs out to a 45-degree angle.

3 Breathe in as you lift the legs up so they are directly over your hips.

4 Breathe out again as you try to bring the feet towards your head, increasing the stretch in the legs.

5 Then breathe in again as you bend your knees, coming back to your starting position.

6 Repeat the whole exercise 6–8 times.

TIPS

- Try to keep your arms and hands relaxed and don't be tempted to push into the floor to help you!
- Keep the core contracted to maintain neutral spine position, avoid allowing the spine to overarch as the legs extend away from your body. If your back is overarching, keep the legs higher than a 45-degree angle until your core strength improves, otherwise you could risk injury to your lower back.
- Keep the movements controlled and the same speed throughout.

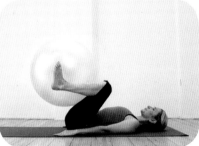

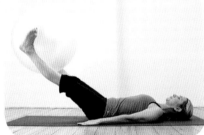

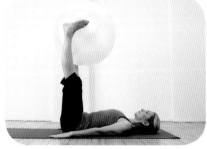

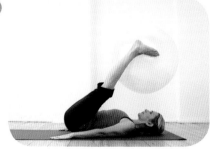

SINGLE LEG STRETCH

? **WHAT FOR?** To gain abdominal strength and to challenge your coordination and breathing!

1 Start lying on your back with your knees bent into your chest and the ball lightly resting on top of your knees.

2 **b** Breathe in to prepare and as you breathe out, reach the ball up above your chest, lift your head a few inches away from the floor and extend your right leg out to a 45-degree angle.

3 **c** Now breathe in as you swap the legs twice, extending first the left and then the right again.

4 **d** Now breathe out again as you swap the legs twice more, but this time take your arms back over your head.

5 Keep breathing in for two leg changes with the arms over your chest.

6 Then breathe out again for two changes with the arms overhead.

7 Repeat this 6–8 times and then bring the arms and knees back into your chest before lowering the legs back to the ground.

TIPS

- The trick with this exercise is to coordinate your breath with the movement, so if it doesn't come easily, don't give up, keep practising! You can also try the legs on their own and then add the arms when you have mastered this, if necessary.
- Be aware of the position of your spine here, making sure that it is staying supported and not arching away from the floor when the arms go overhead.
- If you find this exercise puts too much tension into your neck, try keeping your head rested on the floor.

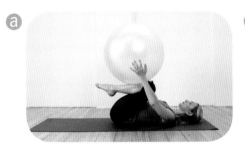

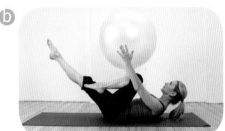

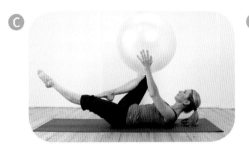

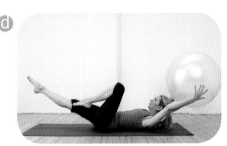

DOUBLE LEG STRETCH

 WHAT FOR? To build abdominal strength and coordination. A really powerful movement.

1 **a** Start lying on your back with your knees bent into your chest and the ball resting on your knees.

2 **b** Breathe in to prepare and as you breathe out, extend the legs away from you to a 45-degree angle. At the same time extend the arms so they are above your forehead.

3 Breathe in as you bring the legs and arms back into the starting position.

4 Repeat this 6–8 times.

TIPS

- When in the extended position think of lengthening through the body, imagine somebody is pulling your head and toes in different directions.
- Keep your legs higher than a 45-degree angle to make this a little easier if necessary. Only lower as far as you are able to stabilise the position of the spine.

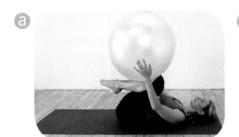

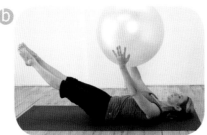

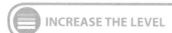 **INCREASE THE LEVEL**

1 **c** Repeat step 1 as before, this time also lifting your head a few inches away from the floor.
2 **d** Repeat step 2 as before, this time extending the arms directly above your head.
3 Repeat steps 3 and 4 as before.

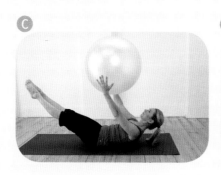

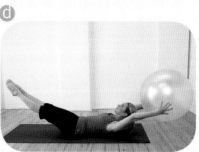

THE ROLL UP

? WHAT FOR? To tone the abdominals and gain core strength. This exercise is for testing core control!

1 **a** Start by lying on your back with your legs extended. Hold the ball lightly on top of your hips.

2 **b** Breathe in and extend your arms up to the ceiling.

3 **c** As you breathe out, curl your body up, peeling the spine away from the floor, one vertebra at a time.

4 **d** Breathe in as you reach the ball towards your feet, stretching as far as you find comfortable.

5 **e** Breathe out again as you curl back down through the spine.

6 **f** Now breathe in as your arms come over your head, reaching towards the wall behind you.

7 Breathe out as you start curling your body up again and repeat the exercise 6–8 times from step 3.

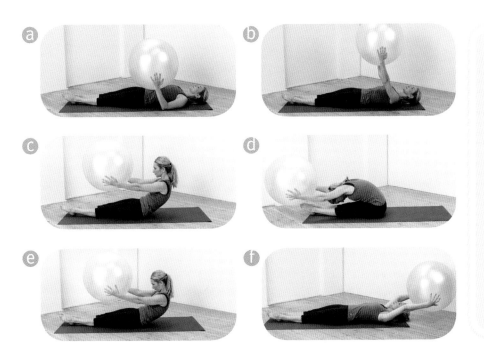

TIPS

- Try to move very slowly and keep at a constant pace throughout. It is very interesting to note where your body wants to speed up and if you can manage to keep control! Really concentrate on the areas where you feel this happening.
- If you find it too hard to lift yourself off the floor with straight legs, try bending your knees until you have more core strength.

THE ROLLOVER

> **?** **WHAT FOR?** To tone the abdominals and legs. This is a very challenging core strength exercise.

1 **a** Start lying on the floor on your back, with the ball between your ankles and your legs extended up towards the ceiling.

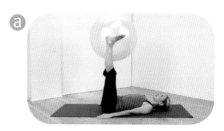

2 **b** Breathe in to prepare and, as you breathe out, roll backwards through the spine taking your legs overhead.

3 Breathe in as you touch the ball on the floor overhead **c** and then lift your legs so they are parallel with the floor. **d**

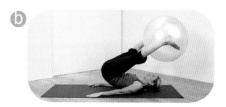

4 **e** Now breathe out as you roll back down through your spine, lowering the ball down to a 45-degree angle.

5 Breathe in again as you bring your legs back to your starting position.

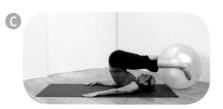

6 Repeat the exercise 4–6 times.

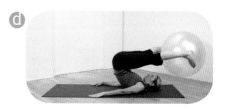

TIPS

- If you find this exercise too challenging, build up strength without the ball and then reintroduce it when you feel ready.
- Keep the exercise slow and steady and at a constant speed throughout.
- When lowering the legs to a 45-degree angle, check that you are able to maintain neutral spine position. Only lower your legs as far as you are able to maintain this, if you feel your lower back starting to arch away from the floor then keep the legs higher until you build core strength.

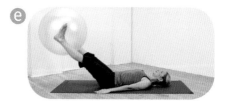

BALL ROLLS

? WHAT FOR? To use the abdominals to control the rolling movement. This is also a great massage for the spine.

1 **(a)** Start balanced on your sitting bones with your knees bent and the ball held in front of your shins.

2 **(b)** Breathe in to prepare, and then breathe out as you round the spine and roll backwards, staying held in your starting position.

3 Breathe in as you roll back up to your starting position and balance here again.

4 Take 6–8 rolls.

TIPS

- Only roll as far as the upper back – your head and neck should not touch the floor.
- Keep your body shape held in the original starting position. The only movement should be the roll. If you go floppy you will find it difficult to roll back up again.

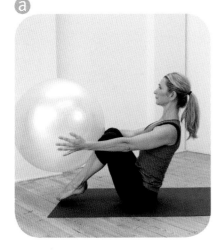

(a)

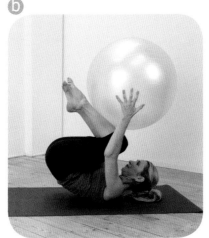

(b)

CHAPTER FIVE

YOGA WITH THE BALL

WHAT IS YOGA?

The word yoga comes from the Sanskrit root 'yuj' which means to join or yoke. It implies the joining of every aspect of a human being: mind, body and soul. Another well used definition of yoga is 'union', meaning the union of the individual spirit with the universe.

Yoga is a 5000-year-old applied science of the mind and body. Practising yoga can help to bring about a balance of the body and mind so that we can maintain an optimum state of health. Yoga does not create health, it creates an internal environment that allows us as individuals to find our own balance. A healthy person is a complete unit of mind, body and spirit. Good health requires a natural diet, fresh air, exercise and an untroubled mind and awareness. Yoga offers this whole philosophy, giving insight into all aspects of life.

The yogis believe that everybody's main goal in life is the search for happiness. They feel that although this is what we all strive to achieve, a significant number of people will continue to settle for brief temporary pleasures. They state that at some point during our spiritual evolution, and over many lives, we will become dissatisfied with these temporary moments and will start on our quest for eternal bliss.

More recently, yoga has also become recognised for its physical benefits and can be accessed in health and fitness centres worldwide. In addition, it has also had a number of celebrity endorsements for its role in creating the perfectly toned body. There are many different styles of yoga, some are more physical and some are more meditative, but they all offer something for everyone.

A SHORT HISTORY OF YOGA

Yoga has been practised in India for over two millennia. There are documented stories and legends testifying to the existence of yoga and to the practitioners associated with it.

Indian literature has a wealth of knowledge about yoga covering every conceivable level. They are, in chronological order: the *Vedas* (books of scriptural knowledge), the *Upanisads* (philosophical speculations), the *Puranas* (ancient cosmologies) and two epics, the *Ramayana* and the *Mahabharata*. The *Mahabharata* contains within it a masterpiece of Indian scripture, called the *Bhagavad Gita*.

Towards the end of the Vedic period there was the aphoristic literature with the 'Yoga Aphorisms' of Patanjali. These are of special interest to yoga students. Patanjali is the legendary founder of yoga. According to tradition he brought to humanity a serenity of spirit through the philosophy of yoga. There are also entire works, both ancient and modern, dealing with yoga philosophy, testifying to the continued relevance of yoga as a discipline.

WHY ADAPT YOGA TO THE BALL?

Adapting yoga to the ball provides a unique mind and body training experience, only made possible by bringing together the balancing qualities of the ball with the postures and focus of yoga. The ball can add a new depth to your yoga practice as the unstable surface offers an added challenge. The stabiliser muscles have to work extremely hard to keep you balanced on the ball and the round surface gives a much wider range of movement, offering ease and adaptability when getting in and out of some of the yoga postures.

For people who are newcomers to yoga, the ball can easily offer a way into some of the postures which otherwise would have required much more strength and agility. The ball gives a way of rolling in and out of some of the positions and supports your body weight when needed. However, use of the ball is not only for those at the beginning of their yoga journey, it can also be used as a tool to intensify movements and increase stretches, adding a new challenge to even the most seasoned yoga student.

THE VITAL BREATH

Breath is synonymous with life. Life enters us on our first inhalation and leaves us on our last. Our breathing is so natural and automatic throughout our lifetime that we mostly don't even notice it is happening, unless our attention is drawn to it through restriction or because we choose to focus our attention on the process.

The practice of consciously controlling the breath – 'Pranayama' – is an ancient tool developed by the yogis ultimately to create harmony in our body, mind and surroundings. The fundamental act of breathing itself creates balance within, by providing the body with a continual supply of new oxygen, while the carbon dioxide we expire is also creating balance to the natural world outside of our body.

In yoga we try to breathe deep into the diaphragm using the full capacity of the lungs. This is the way we were designed to breathe and unfortunately the short shallow breaths that most of us unconsciously rely on do not allow our body to perform at peak efficiency. This seems to have evolved as a consequence of our stressful lifestyles – never really having the opportunity to focus on our breath – and through bad posture – a consequence of our sedentary life choices: car, computer, sofa, TV, bed, etc.

When practising yoga on the ball, we still need to be aware of the breathing techniques we learnt in Chapter 1, pages 24–27, and will need to implement these techniques when in positions on the ball where we need to stabilise the spine to maintain neutral position. However, the following breathing exercise, known as 'diaphragmatic breathing', will draw your attention to breathing deeply and fully with focus, which is our ultimate aim during our yoga practice. This type of breathing is one of a few breathing techniques used in yoga.

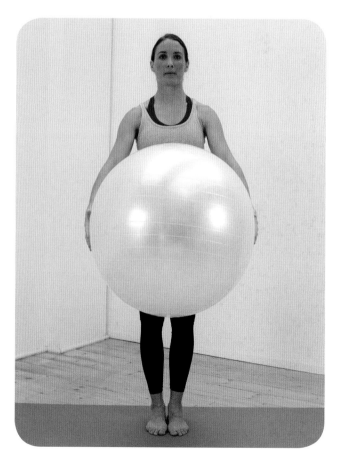

DIAPHRAGMATIC BREATHING EXERCISE

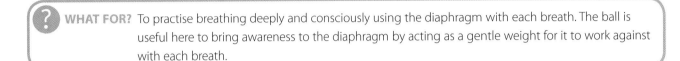

? **WHAT FOR?** To practise breathing deeply and consciously using the diaphragm with each breath. The ball is useful here to bring awareness to the diaphragm by acting as a gentle weight for it to work against with each breath.

1 **a** Start lying on your back with your knees bent up and your feet flat on the floor. Place the ball on your abdomen, keeping your hands on it to secure it.

2 Inhale through your nose, allowing your tummy to swell with the breath, pushing against the ball.

3 Breathe out through the mouth, expelling the air from your lungs, pulling the abdomen in towards your spine.

4 Continue breathing for several minutes.

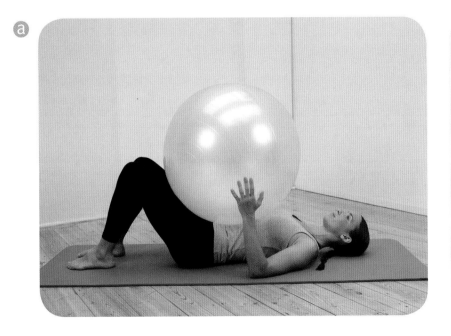

TIPS

- Focus on the movement of the ball as it raises and lowers with each breath.
- Try to make the inhalation and exhalation of your breath the same duration.
- As you settle into your breathing pattern, try to extend the length of each breath.

BREATHING WITH ARM RAISES

? **WHAT FOR?** To continue the deep breathing practice, this time also adding arm raises to master coordination of breath and movement.

1 Start lying on your back with your knees bent up and feet flat on the floor. Place the ball on your abdomen, keeping hold of it with your hands.

2 **a** As you take a breath in, raise the ball up, extending your arms overhead, feeling your tummy swell like a balloon.

3 **b** As you exhale bring the arms back down so the ball is resting once again on your abdomen.

4 Continue breathing for a few minutes.

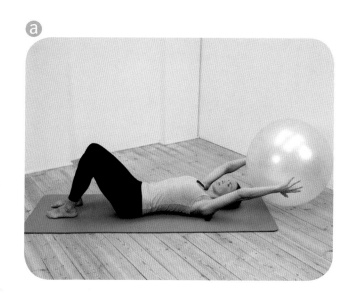

TIPS

- Make sure that as your arms lift overhead you are not allowing your back to arch away from the floor.
- Try to extend the breath, making it last as long as possible.
- Focus on the rise and fall of the tummy even though the ball is now elsewhere.

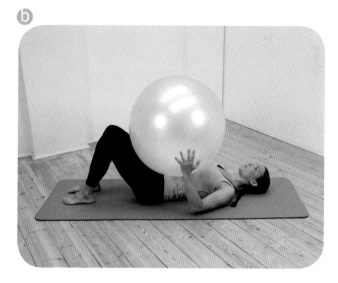

SUN SALUTATION (SALUTE TO THE SUN)

? WHAT FOR? The sun salutation is a yoga-specific warm-up routine designed to lubricate the joints, prepare the muscles, heart, lungs and mind for the more extensive yoga *asanas* to come. This series of movements is to be performed in a continual graceful flow. On days when there is not time for a full yoga practice, this is also an excellent stand-alone routine that you can perform in no time at all. Traditionally this sequence is performed at sunrise to greet the awakening of a new day.

1 **a** Start standing with your feet hip width apart, your knees slightly relaxed, holding the ball in front of you.

2 Breathe in as you raise your straight arms above your head **b** and then sit back into the chair pose. **c**

3 **d** Breathe out as you tilt your body forwards reaching the ball to the floor, keeping extended through the spine. You can bend your knees here if you need to.

4 **e** As you breathe in, place your hands on top of the ball and pull your tummy in, rounding your spine.

5 Breathe out as you walk yourself out onto the ball **f** until you reach the plank posture. **g**

6 **h** Breathe in again as you walk yourself back off the ball, coming into downward-facing dog. Take a few breaths in this position, bending the knees if you need to.

7 **i** As you inhale come down onto your hands, knees over the ball.

8 **j** Breathe out as you push up into cobra, again keeping the knees bent here if necessary.

9 **k** Breathe in again as you lower the body back down onto your hands and knees.

10 **l** Breathe out as you push back up onto your feet, coming back into your forwards tilt.

11 **m** Breathe in as you lift up into the chair pose.

12 **n** Breathe out finally as you straighten your legs and lower the ball back down into your starting position.

13 Repeat the sequence 2–5 times.

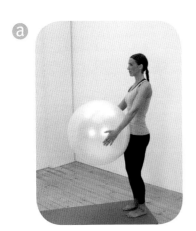

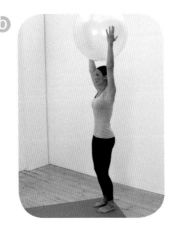

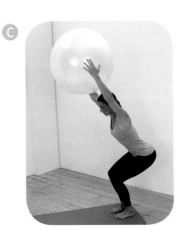

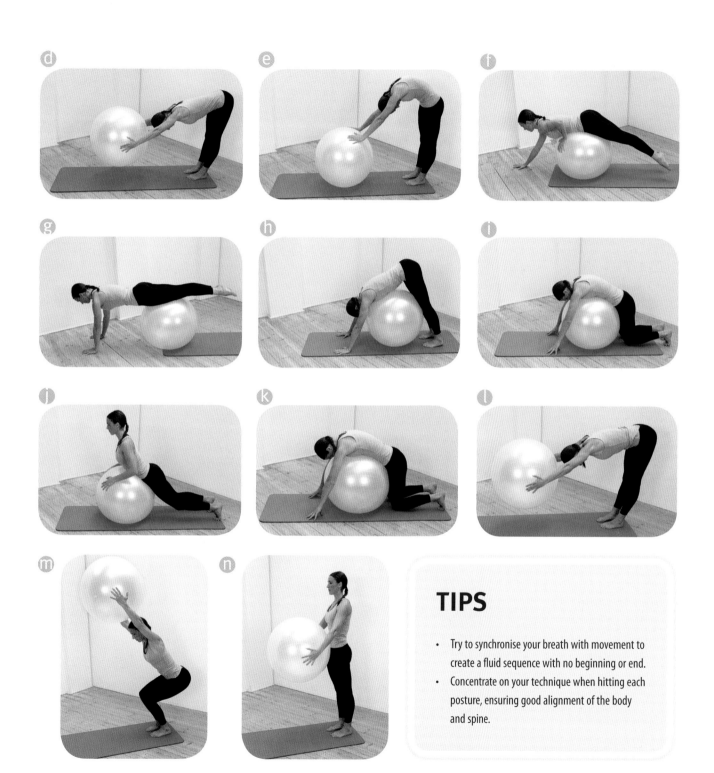

TIPS

- Try to synchronise your breath with movement to create a fluid sequence with no beginning or end.
- Concentrate on your technique when hitting each posture, ensuring good alignment of the body and spine.

STANDING POSTURES

Standing postures are the most fundamental of all the yoga *asanas*, as they pave the way for some of the more advanced postures. These postures create strength, power and confidence as well as increased flexibility and mobility. They can aid digestion, regulate the kidneys and improve circulation, while also invigorating the mind.

Hold each posture as long as is comfortable for you, taking a few deep breaths and coming out when you feel ready.

MOUNTAIN POSE

> **?** **WHAT FOR?** This is used as a starting or finishing position in yoga, but is also very useful to focus your mind and energy before moving into more difficult postures. Use this moment to check alignment and centre yourself.

1 **a** Stand with the ball held in front of you and your arms relaxed down. Make sure that your feet are parallel and your leg muscles are engaged, actively drawing the legs together. Think about drawing your shoulder blades down your back, lift long through the crown of your head and open your chest, lifting your heart.

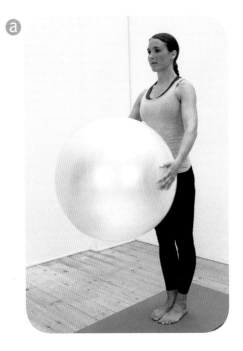

ONE LEG BALANCE

 WHAT FOR? This is a good introductory balance that will warm up the central nervous system and help focus your mind for the more challenging balances to come.

1 **ⓐ** Start standing in front of your ball, place your right foot onto the ball.

2 **ⓑ** Stand up tall and bring your arms down by your sides.

3 Breathe deeply while balancing here.

4 When you are ready come out of the balance and swap to the other leg.

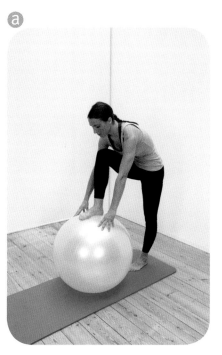

ⓐ

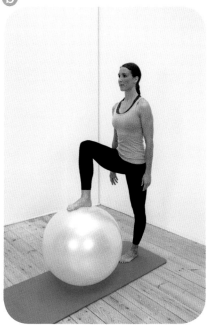

ⓑ

TIPS

- Try to find a point at eye level to focus on. This will help you to maintain your balance.
- Connect your core muscles at the beginning of the sequence. This will keep you strong and controlled.

SIDE BEND

? WHAT FOR? To open up your lungs and increase flexibility down each side.

1 **a** Start standing tall with your feet hip width apart and the ball held above your head.

2 **b** Grow tall, then breathe out as you reach the ball towards the right side, bending the upper body as far as is comfortable.

3 Take a few breaths here and then return to standing, lengthening further as you come up. Repeat on the other side.

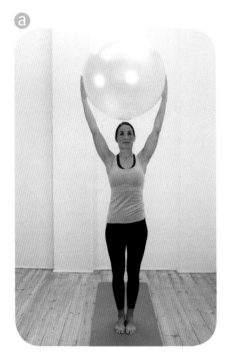

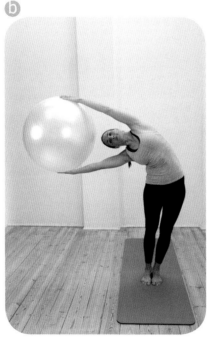

TIPS

- Keep your hips and shoulders square on to the front as you bend.
- Keep your head in line with the rest of the spine as you bend. Try not to carry too much tension in the neck.
- Imagine growing taller each time you return to the centre.

FORWARD FOLD

? **WHAT FOR?** To strengthen the back and backs of the legs, and to increase flexibility in these areas. This is also good for practising maintaining neutral spine posture while folding forwards.

1 **a** Start standing with the ball held in front of you.

2 **b** Breathe out as you fold forwards from the hips, keeping the spine extended, reaching the ball towards the floor.

3 Take a few deep breaths here.

4 Breathe in as you return to your starting position.

a
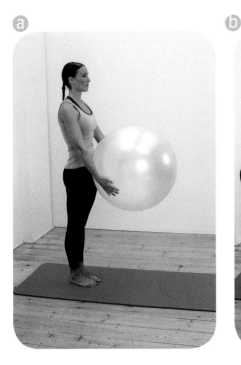

b
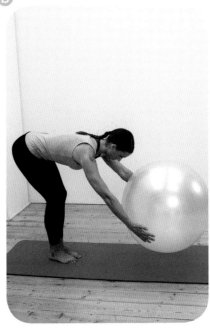

TIPS

- Fold as far as is comfortable for your body.
- Keep an extended neutral spine position throughout.
- Keep the knee joints slightly relaxed in this position.

CHAIR POSE

> **?** **WHAT FOR?** To strengthen the muscles in the legs and arms and to open up the back. This *asana* also stimulates the digestive and reproductive systems.

1 **a** Start standing tall with your feet hip width apart and the ball held in front of your legs.

2 **b** Breathe out as you sit back (just like you are sitting into a chair), reaching the ball down towards the floor.

3 Take some breaths here, then straighten the legs coming back to your starting position.

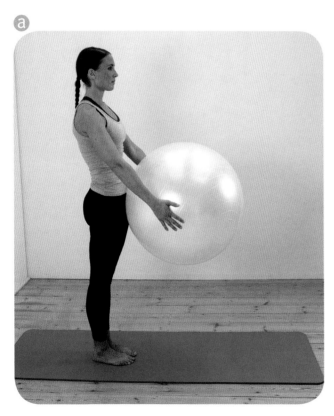

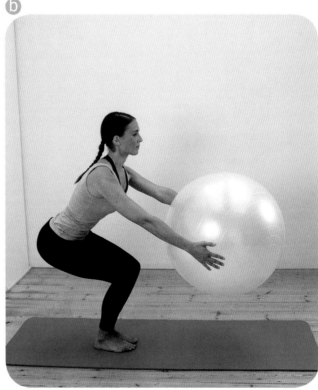

1 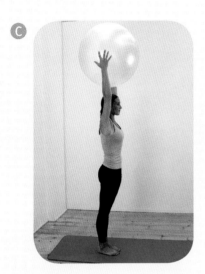 Start standing as before, but this time with the ball held above your head

2 Breathe out as you sit back, keeping the arms reaching towards the ceiling.

3 Repeat step 3 as before.

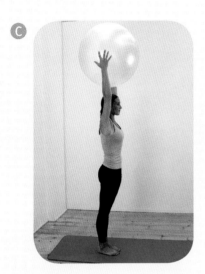

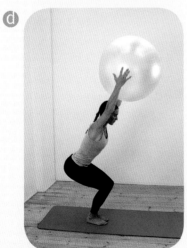

TIPS

- Keep your knees in line with, and directly over, your ankles as you sit back into Chair Pose.
- If it feels like there is too much pressure on your knees, take a gentler version by not bending so deeply into the pose.
- Keep a feeling of lift in your chest throughout.

PYRAMID POSE

? WHAT FOR? To increase flexibility in the backs of the legs and the lower back.

1 **a** Start standing with the ball on the floor in front of you and your hands resting on top of the ball.

2 **b** Step your right leg back and turn the foot out to a 45-degree angle. Bend your left knee, making sure your hips are square on to the front.

3 **c** Breathe out and roll the ball away from you at the same time as extending your left knee.

4 Hold the pose, taking a few deep breaths here. When you are ready, come out of the position and then repeat on the other side.

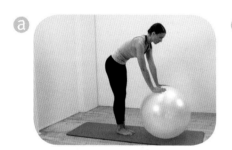
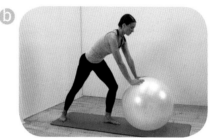
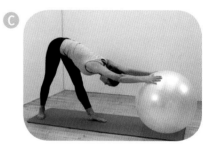

INCREASE THE LEVEL

1 Repeat steps 1–3 as before.
2 **d** Once in the pose we are going to add a spinal twist. Reach your right arm up towards the ceiling, looking up at the right hand.
3 Repeat step 4 as before, then repeat on the other side.

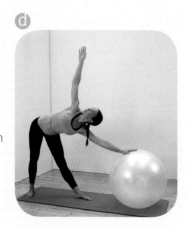

TIPS

- Use the ball to increase or decrease the stretch by rolling it in or out to suit your flexibility.
- When in the pose make sure that your spine is extended rather than rounded.
- Allow yourself to relax into the stretch, taking deep breaths. You should find that as the muscles relax you can move a bit deeper into the posture.

WARRIOR 1

? WHAT FOR? To strengthen the front of the thighs and tone all the smaller stabiliser muscles of the legs. This will also stretch the hips and shoulders as well as aid digestion and circulation.

1 **a** Start standing tall with the ball held in front of your legs in Mountain Pose (see page 166).

2 **b** Step your right leg forwards one comfortable stride's length, then turn your left foot out to a 45-degree angle.

3 **c** Bend your right knee, coming into a lunge position and reach the ball up above your head.

4 Stay here for a few breaths then, when you are ready, come out of the posture and repeat on the other leg.

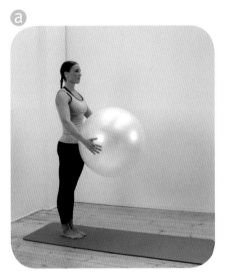

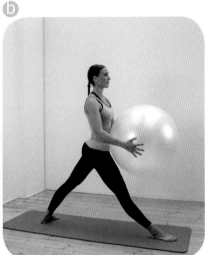

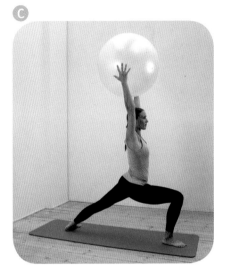

TIPS

- Make sure your bent supporting knee stays over the line of your ankle in Warrior 1. If you need to, step the back leg further out to achieve this.
- Lengthening tall as you reach the arms towards the ceiling will aid balance and stability when in the full posture.

WARRIOR 2

? **WHAT FOR?** This strong posture strengthens and tones the legs and stretches the inner thigh muscles. The great benefit of using the ball here is that you can actually make it a seated posture as a beginner's version, progressing to standing when you feel ready.

1 **(a)** Start seated on your ball with your legs wide. Reach your arms out to the sides at shoulder height.

2 **(b)** Turn your left foot out and your right foot in. Push yourself forwards onto the edge of the ball, extending your right leg and looking forwards over the line of your left hand.

3 Hold for a few breaths then repeat on the other side.

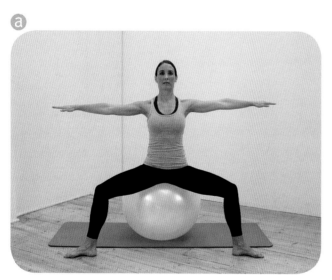

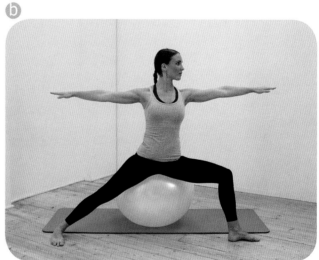

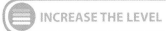
1 c Start in Mountain Pose (see page 166) with the ball held in front of your legs.
2 d Step your legs out wide to the sides and place the ball on your left hip, keeping it in place by resting your left arm on top. Take the right arm out to the side also.
3 e Turn your left foot out and your right foot in and bend your left knee to a 90-degree angle. Look forwards over your left hand.
4 Hold for a few breaths then repeat on the other side.

c

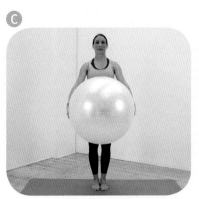

d

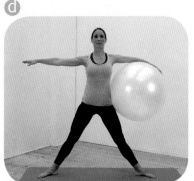

e

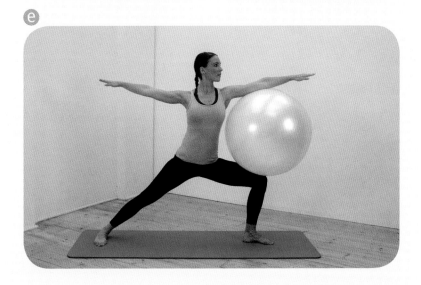

TIPS

- When taking the seated version of Warrior 2, use the ball to support you as much or as little as you need. Try taking your weight right to the edge of the ball and lift from your legs so you are barely in contact with the ball. Once you can manage this you know you are ready to move on to the next level.
- In both versions of the posture, make sure that the supporting bent knee is lined up directly over the line of the ankle. This will avoid putting too much pressure onto the knee joint.
- Think of lengthening long through the fingertips as if you are being pulled in opposite directions.

POSE OF THE DANCER

> **? WHAT FOR?** To practise your balancing skills and to tone and strengthen the stabiliser muscles in the legs and increase core strength.

1   Start standing with the ball placed on the floor in front of you. Place your feet together, bend your knees and rest your hands lightly on top of the ball.

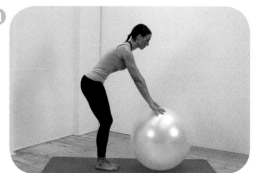

2   Take hold of your right foot with your right hand behind your back, bringing your knees together and contracting your core muscles to aid balance.

3   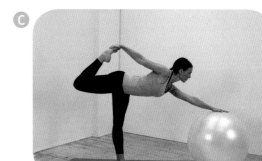 Now tilt forwards from your hips, rolling the ball out with your left hand as far as you can.

4   Try and balance here while you take a few breaths, then roll the ball back in to come out of the pose. Repeat on the other side.

TIPS

- Make sure the spine stays extended as you tilt the body forwards.
- Find a point at eye level to focus on throughout the exercise as this will help you concentrate and aid balance.
- Only tilt as far as you feel comfortable to start with. Building balance and strength over time will enable you to progress into the full position.

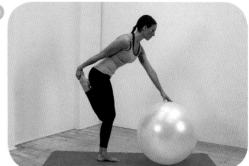

WARRIOR 3

? WHAT FOR? This last posture from the Warrior series is a more advanced posture. It will tone and strengthen the legs and core muscles and will test your balancing skills, helping to ground and centre you.

1 Start by standing tall in Mountain Pose (see page 166). **a**

2 Now extend your right leg behind you and lift your ball forwards to shoulder height. **b**

3 Tilt forwards from the hips, aiming to come to a straight line from your hands through to your right foot. **c**

4 Take a few breaths balancing here. When you are ready, bring yourself out of the posture and repeat on the other side.

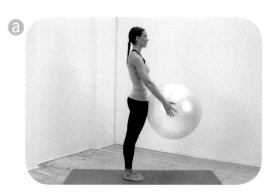

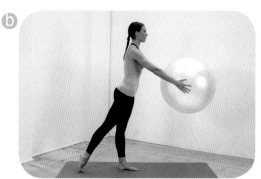

TIPS

- If you find this difficult, start by only taking yourself halfway into the desired position. You will soon build confidence and balance skills, enabling you to master the full posture.
- Keep focused on a fixed point at floor level in front of you. This will help you to stay focused and balanced.
- Think again of a lengthening through the body; imagine your arms and working leg being pulled apart in opposite directions.

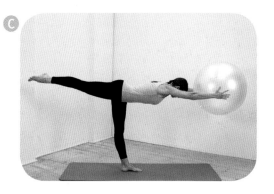

POSTURES ON AND UNDER THE BALL

The following postures are going to utilise the ball in a slightly different way. We will be using it to sit on, roll over, lift and to modify some of these traditional yoga postures. Challenge yourself with each of the postures, but find what Buddha referred to as 'the middle way' – a compromise between challenge and comfort. Only you know your own body, so do what's right for you and use your ball as a support when needed or a tool to increase intensity when it feels right. Again, hold each posture as long as feels right for your body, breathing deeply throughout.

TEMPLE POSE

WHAT FOR? To stretch the inner thigh muscles and loosen up the hips. This is also a good opportunity to tune in to your balancing skills on the ball.

1 a Start seated on the ball with your legs out wide and your knees and feet turned out to a 45-degree angle.

2 b Place the palms of your hands together into prayer position and then push your hips forwards on the ball, increasing the stretch. Take a few breaths here for as long as you are comfortable.

TIPS

- Your weight should be right at the front of your ball, enabling you to fully open up your hips as far as your flexibility will allow.
- Connect your core muscles and focus on a fixed spot in front of you to help you stay balanced on the ball.

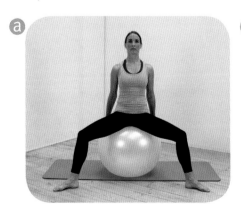

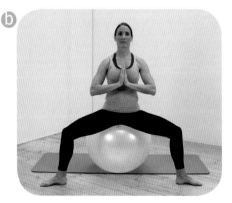

FAN POSTURE

? WHAT FOR? To stretch through the chest, shoulders and upper back. This posture really gives you a sense of opening up the lungs.

1 Start seated on the ball with your feet out wide, place your hands on the floor between your feet and relax your body over. Ensure that your hips are directly over the line of your feet throughout the posture.

2 **b** Now push back on your ball, extending your legs as far as you can, and extend your arms so that your body is parallel with the floor.

3 **c** Adjust your right hand so it is directly underneath your nose, and now reach your left hand up towards the ceiling, looking towards your fingers.

4 Take some breaths in this position, and then relax both arms back to the floor before repeating on the other side.

TIPS

- Connect your core muscles by pulling your navel in towards your spine. This will keep the spine supported throughout the rotation.
- Think about opening up through the chest and lifting towards the ceiling.

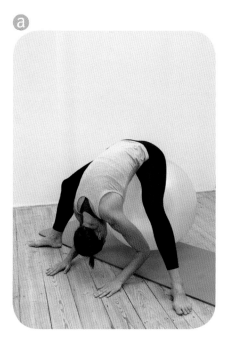

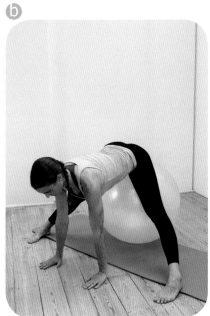

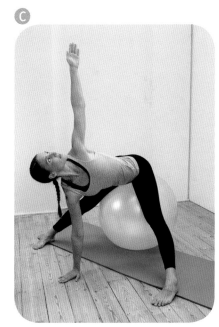

TREE POSE

1 **ⓐ** Start seated on the ball with your feet hip width apart and your arms relaxed down by your sides.

2 **ⓑ** Now lift your right foot off the floor and place the sole of the foot against your left ankle.

3 **ⓒ** Keeping your balance, float the arms up towards the ceiling, and then bring them down in front of your chest into prayer position.

4 Take some breaths in this position and then repeat on the other leg.

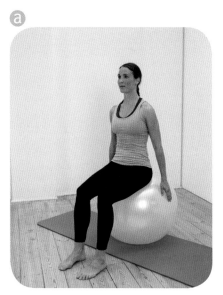

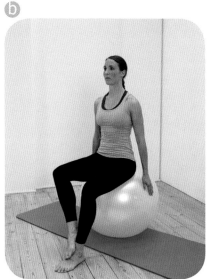

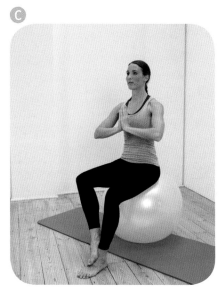

1 Repeat step 1 as before.
2 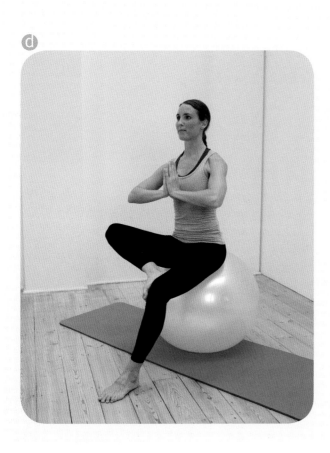 Lift your right foot off the floor and place the sole of the foot against your left knee. Now float the arms up into prayer position as before.
3 Repeat step 4 as before.

TIPS

- Focus on a fixed point in front of you to aid balance.
- If you need to, keep your arms by your sides until you have gained confidence in your balancing skills.

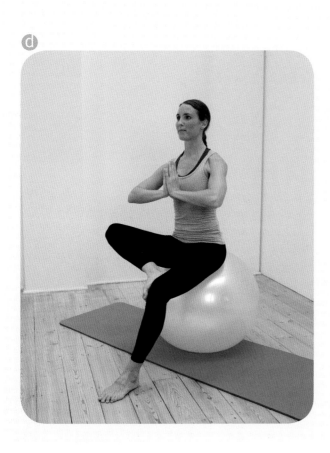

CROW POSE

1 Start seated on your ball with your feet hip width apart and your knees bent. Rest your hands lightly on the ball for support.

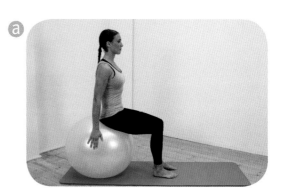

2 **b** Walk yourself out on the ball, allowing it to roll up your spine. Stop when it is resting in your lower back. Drop your hips towards the floor and wrap your arms around the ball behind you.

3 **c** Now lift your hips and lie back into a table top position.

4 Hold the posture while you take a few deep breaths.

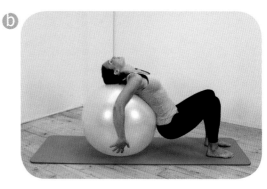

TIPS

• Align your shoulders, hips and knees when in Crow Pose.
• Also align your knees directly over your ankles.

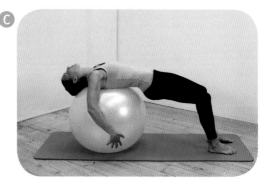

THE CAT

> **? WHAT FOR?** This exercise is a fantastic warm up for the spine, great for releasing any pent up tension. It is also a really useful exercise for practising coordination of your breath and movement, as the movement really makes sense of the breathing pattern.

1 **a** Start on your hands and knees on the floor with the ball underneath your torso.

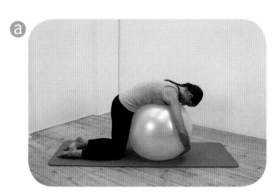

2 **b** Breathe out as you curve the spine and drop the head forwards.

3 **c** Breathe in as you lift your head and slightly arch into the lower back.

4 Alternate between these two movements 6–8 times, or as long as is comfortable.

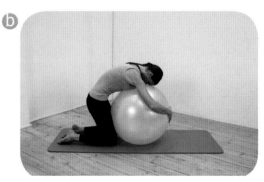

TIPS

- Ensure that your knees are directly underneath your hips and your hands are under your shoulders.
- Get into a rhythm with the movements and your breath, trying to elongate the breath as much as possible.
- Use the ball to curl around and push against as the torso moves.

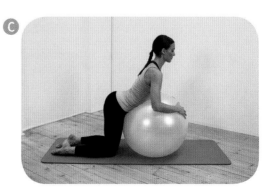

THREAD THE NEEDLE

? **WHAT FOR?** This is a fantastic stretch for the upper back and the shoulders.

1 Start kneeling up in front of your ball with your hands placed lightly on top.

2 **b** Roll the ball away from you until your arms are extended and your torso is parallel with the floor.

3 **c** Thread your right arm underneath your body as far as is comfortable, allowing your upper back to twist.

4 Hold the position while you take a few breaths and then release. Repeat on the other side.

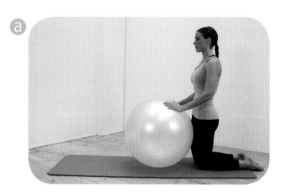

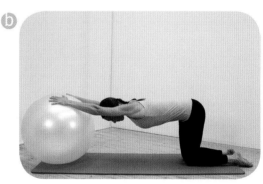

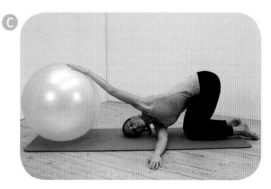

TIPS

- Make sure before you start that your knees are aligned underneath your hips.
- Keep the back in an extended position as you thread the arm underneath yourself.
- Turn to look towards the underneath arm, keeping the neck in line with the rest of the spine.

DOWNWARD DOG

? WHAT FOR? To strengthen your chest, arms, shoulders and thigh muscles, as well as giving a stretch to the chest, shoulders and backs of your legs. This will also encourage a lengthening through the spine.

1 **a** Start on your hands and knees over the ball.

2 **b** Curl your toes underneath and push your bottom towards the ceiling extending your legs. Push your heels towards the floor and your chest into the ball.

3 Hold this posture for a few breaths until you need to relax.

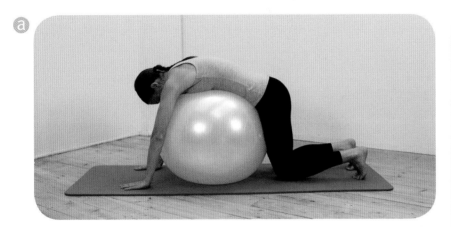

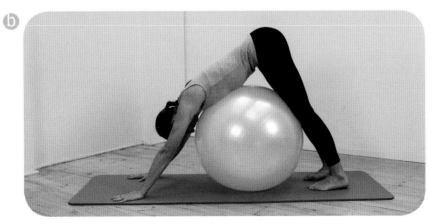

TIPS

- Keep the spine lengthened.
- Keep a feeling of length going through the legs, pushing the heels into the floor.
- Imagine someone's hand between your shoulder blades applying pressure. This should encourage the chest to push towards the ball.

BOAT POSE

 WHAT FOR? To strengthen and tone the abdominal muscles.

1   Start seated on the floor with your feet resting on the ball and your hands on the floor just behind your bottom.

2 Now place your feet either side of the ball, gripping it between your ankles. Lift your arms, reach them towards your feet and tilt your torso back so you are leaning away from the ball.

3 Hold this posture for a few breaths and then relax.

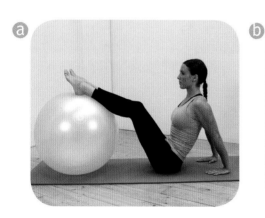

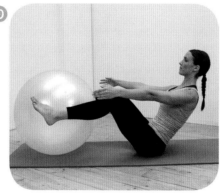

TIPS

- Do not allow the spine to curve as you tilt the torso back.
- If you would like to increase the level of this posture further, try straightening the legs once they are lifted.

 INCREASE THE LEVEL

1 Repeat step 1 as before.
2 Repeat step 2, but this time lift the ball off the floor until your feet come level with your knees.
3 Repeat step 3 as before.

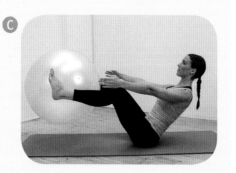

COBRA

1 **ⓐ** Start on your hands and knees over the ball.

2 **ⓑ** Place your hands onto the ball, curl your toes underneath you, engage your core muscles and then lift your torso away from the ball.

3 Hold the posture for a few breaths and then relax back down.

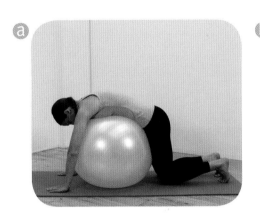

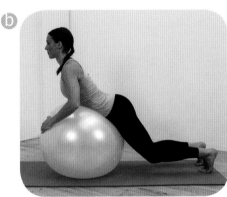

TIPS

- Keep your core muscles engaged throughout to avoid overarching the lower back.
- Think of lifting the chest towards the ceiling, giving a feeling of opening out.

 INCREASE THE LEVEL

1 Repeat step 1 as before.
2 **ⓒ** Repeat step 2, this time fully extending your legs.
3 Repeat step 3 as before.

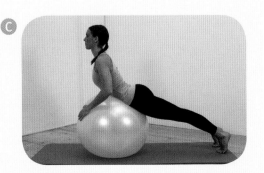

CANDLE POSE

? WHAT FOR? To strengthen your abdominal muscles as well as improving your balance skills.

1 **ⓐ** Start lying on your back with your knees bent, feet flat on the floor and the ball held between your ankles.

2 **ⓑ** Breathe in to prepare then, as you breathe out, raise the feet off the floor, bringing your knees in towards your chest.

3 **ⓒ** Place your hands underneath you on your hip bones and let them support you as you lift your hips off the floor, aligning your hips directly above your elbows.

4 Try to hold this posture for a few breaths then gently lower yourself down.

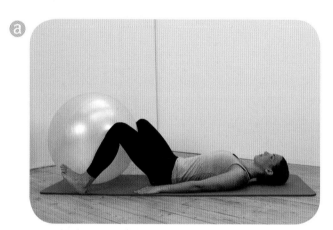

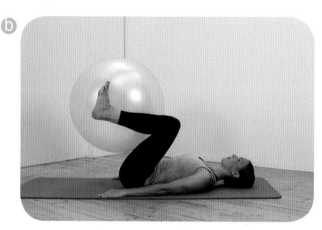

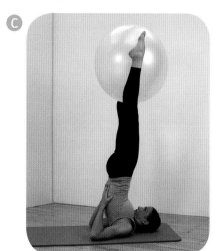

TIPS

- Make sure that you are not taking any of your weight back into your neck.
- The ball should be aligned over your chest.

SIDE PLANK

? WHAT FOR? This is a strong posture for gaining core strength and improving balance.

1 **a** Start kneeling up with the ball by your right side.

2 **b** Reach your right arm over the ball and place the hand onto the floor. Once you have done this, extend your left leg out to the side.

3 **c** Reach your left arm towards the ceiling and extend your right leg, placing the feet together. Look up towards your extended arm.

4 Hold this posture for a few breaths.

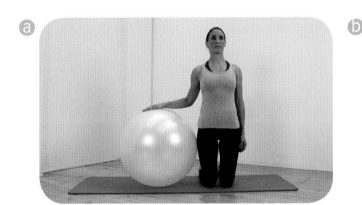

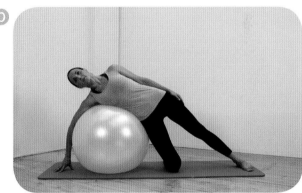

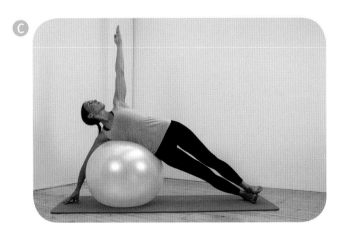

TIPS

- Try to integrate the body here into one solid piece. As soon as any part of the body relaxes you will start to wobble!
- Try not to allow too much tension to creep into the neck.

REVERSE PLANK

? WHAT FOR? This is a more advanced posture, good for developing core stability as well as strengthening your arms and shoulders.

1 Start sitting on the floor with your feet resting on top of the ball, your knees slightly bent and your hands resting on the floor behind you, fingers pointing away from your body.

2 **b** Breathe out as you lift your bottom a few inches away from the floor.

3 Hold this position for a few breaths.

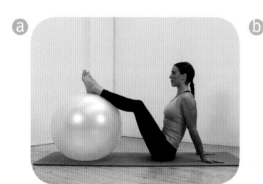

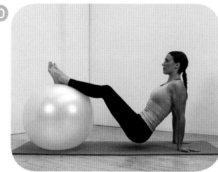

INCREASE THE LEVEL

1 Repeat step 1 as before.
2 **c** As you breathe out, lift your bottom off the floor until your body is in a straight line parallel to the floor.
3 Hold for a few deep breaths.

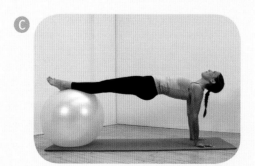

TIPS

- Keep the connection in your core active while holding the posture.
- Make sure that the weight of your body is distributed evenly between your hands.
- Keep your neck in line with the rest of your spine, with your chin lifted away from your chest.

BOW POSE

 WHAT FOR? To strengthen your lower back and buttocks, as well as offering a lovely stretch to the chest and the front of the thighs.

1 ⓐ Start lying on the floor on your front with the ball held between your ankles. Have your arms relaxed by your sides.

2 ⓑ Engage your core muscles and breathe out as you lift the upper body away from the floor, reaching behind you with your arms. Simultaneously bend your knees, bringing the ball closer to your bottom.

3 Hold the posture while you take a few deep breaths, then relax.

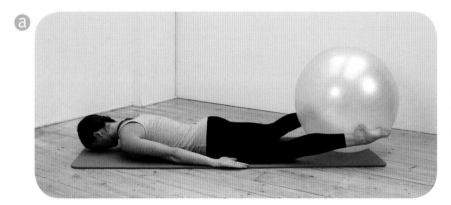

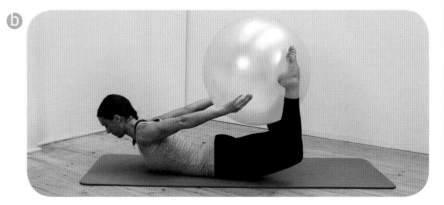

TIPS

- Keep your core contracted throughout to avoid overarching the back.
- Keep lengthened through the back of the neck, maintaining alignment with the rest of the spine.
- Try not to let your breathing become shallow or laboured.

RELAXATION POSTURES

These postures offer a rest from physical activity and can be performed at the end of your yoga practice as a cool down, as well as a chance to relax and increase mental clarity. The postures can also be used throughout your practice whenever a rest is needed. Take time in these positions to embrace the sensations they provide and to focus on your breathing.

If you would like to take your relaxation further into a full meditation, see the meditation exercises in Chapter 9, pages 270–275. If you would like further muscle specific stretches to increase flexibility see Chaper 6, page 198–217.

POSE OF THE CHILD

? WHAT FOR? This is a modified version of a well-used relaxation posture for the ball. This position is great for releasing tension in the spine and throughout the entire body. This is the position we may have come to as children when in need of comfort.

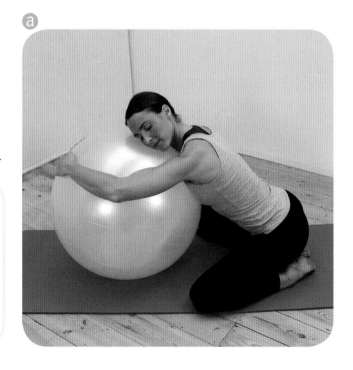

1 **ⓐ** Start kneeling on the floor in front of your ball. Relax forwards, allowing your body to drape over the ball. Adjust your legs so that your knees are apart and your feet touching.

2 Stay relaxed in this position, allowing yourself to rock backwards and forwards on the ball to adjust the position if you wish. Stay relaxed for as long as you need.

TIPS

- Allow your body to mould around the ball in the way that feels most appropriate and comfortable to you.
- Focus on your breathing when in the position, allowing your tension to seep away.

CORPSE POSE

? WHAT FOR? This is the quintessential restorative pose used for deep relaxation and rejuvenation. Quite often the final posture in your practice.

1 **a** Start lying on your back with your heels resting up on the ball, arms relaxed by your sides.

2 Focus on your breath, taking deep diaphragmatic breaths.

3 Stay here for as long as your schedule allows.

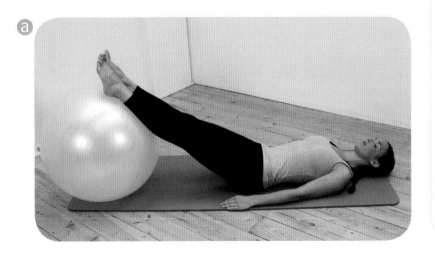

TIP

- Allow your body to relax fully in this position so that there is complete stillness throughout.

CHAPTER SIX

BALL STRETCHES

INTRODUCTION

I find stretching the most deliciously satisfying way to release tension from my body. I love the slightly uncomfortable feeling of muscular tension when I first move into a stretch and then how the muscle extends like a piece of elastic and the pain starts to drift away. Add a ball into the mix and you have something firm and yet comfortable to drape yourself over in any direction, giving you more ways to stretch than ever. You can use the rolling motion of the ball to gracefully roll in and out of each position as well as easily control the intensity of your stretch.

It constantly surprises me that so many people seem to neglect this important and enjoyable component of their sport or fitness training. When I have asked personal clients why this is, it seems that many people believe it can't have any real benefits as it is not an element of their training that causes them to be out of breath and sweaty.

Stretching is an important element of any programme. Not only should it be used to increase your flexibility and maintain mobility in later life, it should also form part of your warm-up routine to minimise your risk of injury, as well as your cool-down routine at the end of each workout to reduce post-exercise muscle soreness.

There are three main types of stretches; you will need to choose the right type of stretch depending on whether you are warming up, cooling down or trying to increase your flexibility.

STATIC STRETCHES

A static stretch is mostly used to maintain flexibility and is where you move in to a stretch and hold for a predetermined amount of time – usually around 10–20 seconds. If you breathe deeply and relax into the stretch, you will find that after about 15 seconds your muscles relax as the body's natural inhibitor switches off. You will feel that you can suddenly move a little deeper into the position.

DEVELOPMENTAL STRETCHES

This is the same as a static stretch, except the intention is to increase flexibility. Each stretch is therefore held for longer – usually between 30–60 seconds – allowing the muscles time to relax and then extend. Developmental stretching can also be executed with help from another person – this is sometimes called assisted stretching. Your assistant can gradually apply pressure to the muscle, helping to increase the stretch. This should be done carefully with constant communication from the person being stretched!

DYNAMIC STRETCHES

This type of stretching is usually seen as part of a warm-up routine. The purpose is not to increase flexibility, but to prepare the muscles for the work to come as well as to mobilise the joints. Some examples of this type of stretching would be arm circles, leg swings or lunges. The aim would be to gradually increase the range of movement over 10–15 repetitions. This type of stretching is performed in a steady rhythmical motion so that the heart rate stays elevated and your muscles stay warm. You will find these exercises as part of the warm-up section in Chapter 1, pages 28–47.

STRETCHING FOR A BRIGHTER FUTURE

There is one last very important reason why you should make stretching a part of your routine. The benefits will stay with you into your later years and can have an astonishing effect on your quality of life. When you think about the challenges that elderly people face, quite often you will find that the most difficult is the loss of independence caused by limited mobility and flexibility. This can have a knock-on effect, lowering confidence and leading to disempowerment.

The trouble is, once we stop doing some of these physical tasks for ourselves we quickly lose strength and mobility and find ourselves on a rapid downward spiral. The key is, where possible, to maintain confidence in our functional fitness. We can increase our chances of this by ensuring we remain mobile and flexible, which assists us in carrying out everyday tasks.

The ball is easy to store in the corner of the room and is great for pulling out while watching your favourite 'soap' and enjoying a few stretches. There has never been a more accessible way to make this a part of your life.

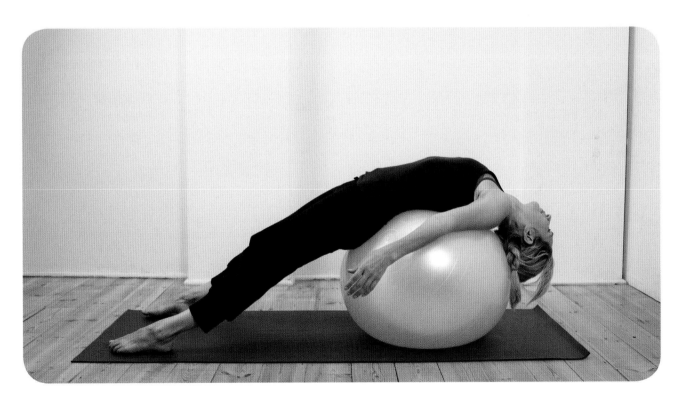

UPPER BODY STRETCHES

BALL SIDE BEND

? **WHAT FOR?** A stretch for the side of the body, using the weight of the ball to increase intensity.

1 Start standing with your feet hip width apart and the ball held above your head.

2 Bend your body towards the right side as far as you can, keeping the hips square on to the front.

3 Hold the stretch for up to 20 seconds and then come back to the centre. Repeat on the left side.

TIPS

- Think of lengthening tall so your body stays elongated as you bend to the side. You can grow even taller each time you return to the centre.
- Keep your hips and shoulders square on to the front throughout the bend.
- Try to keep your neck in alignment with the rest of the spine.

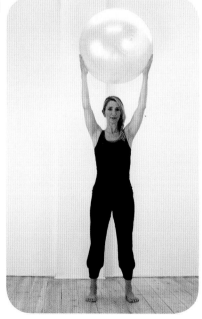

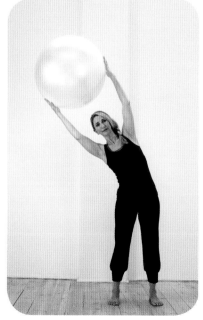

STANDING CAT STRETCH

? **WHAT FOR?** This is a lovely stretch and release for the upper back.

1 **a** Start standing with your feet hip width apart, the ball placed on the floor in front of you and your hands placed on top of the ball. Your back should be in a flattened position.

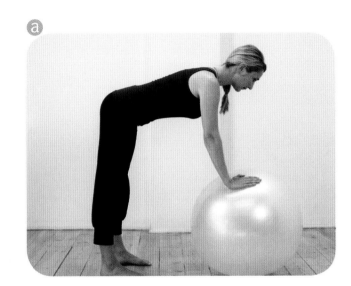

2 **b** Breathe out as you round the upper back, until you feel a stretch down the spine.

3 Hold the stretch for up to 10 seconds and then release back to your starting position. Repeat 3–5 times.

TIPS

- Tuck your head into your chest as you round the back so the stretch reaches all the way up to your neck.
- Ensure that you find your neutral spine position as you return to the centre between each stretch.

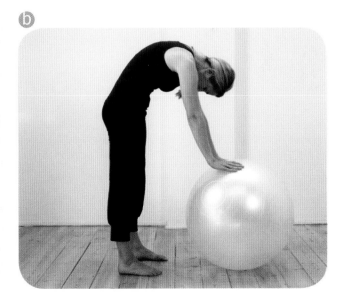

STANDING BACK STRETCH

? WHAT FOR? To stretch the muscles of the shoulders and the upper back.

1 **a** Start standing with your feet hip width apart and the ball placed on the floor in front of you. Place your right hand on the ball with your thumb facing up and your left hand behind your back.

2 **b** Roll the ball away from you and then with your right hand move it towards the left side as far as you can, whilst still keeping your hips square on to the front.

3 Hold the stretch for up to 10 seconds and then repeat on the other side.

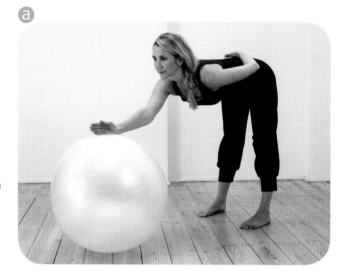

TIPS

- Keep your hips and shoulders square on to the front. The only movement happening should be from your arm.
- Keep your spine in a flat position throughout.

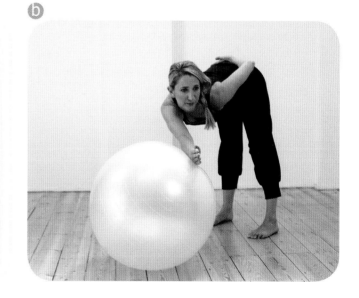

SEATED TRICEP STRETCH

? WHAT FOR? To stretch the tricep muscles in the backs of the arms.

1 **a** Start seated on the ball with your feet hip width apart.

2 **b** Reach your right arm up above your head and then drop your hand down your back as far as possible. Use your left hand to apply pressure to your elbow to increase the stretch.

3 Hold the stretch for up to 10 seconds and then repeat on the other side.

TIPS

- Start seated tall and keep the spine lengthened throughout.
- If you want to increase the stretch slightly, reach your left hand up your back and link fingers with your right hand to apply the pressure.

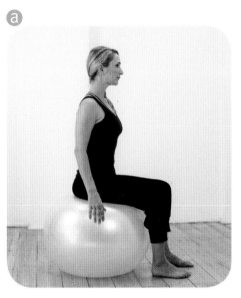

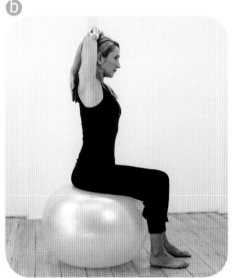

KNEELING CHEST STRETCH

? WHAT FOR? A great stretch for the chest and shoulders. Use the rolling motion of the ball to adjust the intensity to suit you.

1 **a** Start kneeling up, knees hip width apart, with the ball on the floor in front of you and your hands placed on top of the ball.

2 **b** Roll the ball out until your spine is lengthened, and then push your chest towards the floor.

3 Hold this stretch for up to 20 seconds and then relax.

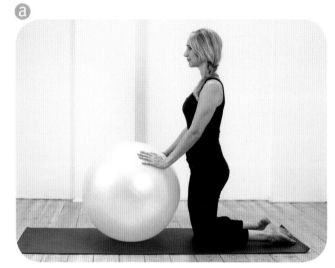

TIPS

- Think of opening up through the chest and shoulders as you ease the chest towards the floor.
- Keep your core contracted to avoid overarching the spine as you stretch.

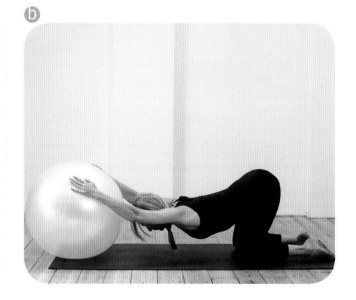

LYING CHEST STRETCH

? WHAT FOR? This is one of my favourite stretching exercises on the ball. It gives a real feeling of opening up in the chest and leaves you feeling re-energised.

1 **a** Start seated on the ball with your feet hip width apart.

2 **b** Walk your feet out, allowing the ball to roll up your spine. Stop when the ball is underneath your lower back.

3 **c** Drop your hips towards the floor and rest your head back on the ball.

4 **d** Now, holding this position, roll yourself back slightly on the ball until your chest is facing the ceiling. Open your arms out to the sides.

5 Hold this stretch for up to 20 seconds and reverse the process to come out of it.

TIP

- If you want to increase this stretch further you can try holding light weights in your hands to add intensity to the stretch across the chest.

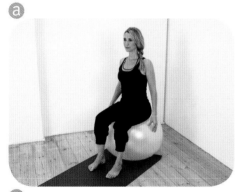

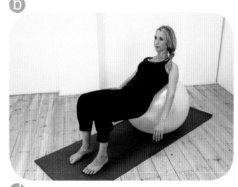

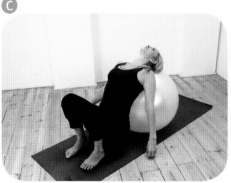

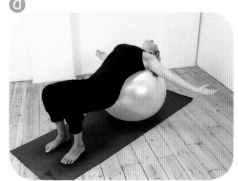

SPINE TWIST

? **WHAT FOR?** To stretch the lower back, increasing flexibility.

1 **a** Start lying on your back with the ball placed on the floor and your lower legs resting on top of the ball. Keep your arms relaxed out to the sides.

2 **b** Allow your knees to roll over to the right side as far as you can, keeping both shoulders pushed into the floor.

3 Hold the stretch for as long as is comfortable – up to a minute, and then come back to the centre. Repeat on the other side.

TIPS

- Control the movement as the knees drop over to one side. You can use the ball to easily roll the legs over and then back up.
- Try looking towards your left hand as your legs roll over to the right to increase the stretch across the spine. Look right when your legs roll to the left.

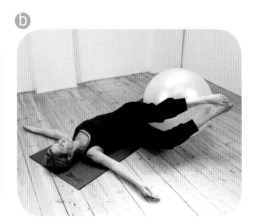

a **b**

LOWER BODY STRETCHES

SEATED HAMSTRING STRETCH

? WHAT FOR? To stretch and increase flexibility in the hamstrings and to stretch the calf muscles.

1 **ⓐ** Start seated on the ball with your feet hip width apart.

2 **ⓑ** Extend your right leg, placing your heel into the floor, rest your hands onto your left thigh and then tilt your body forwards, keeping your right leg extended.

3 Hold this stretch for between 30–60 seconds. Repeat on the other side.

TIPS

- Keep your chest lifted as you tilt forwards so that the spine stays extended.
- Try to keep the knee slightly relaxed so you don't lock into the joint.
- The further you can lower the body over, the more you will increase the stretch.

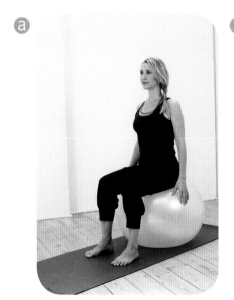

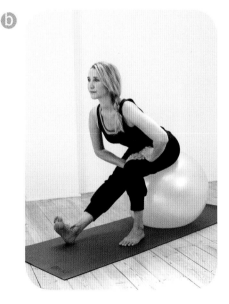

LUNGE STRETCH

? WHAT FOR? This is a strong stretch for the hip flexor and the front of the thighs. Use the ball to take some of your weight if you need to.

1 **a** Start standing with the ball placed on the floor in front of you and your hands resting on top of the ball.

2 **b** Step your left foot to the left of the ball and send your right leg back into a lunge, guiding the ball so it is underneath your right hip.

3 Hold the stretch here for up to 20 seconds. Repeat on the other side.

TIPS

- Ensure that your back leg is extended when in the lunge position.
- Use the ball underneath your hip as much or as little as you need.
- If you would like to increase the intensity of the stretch, roll the ball further up the body so that it is underneath your torso.

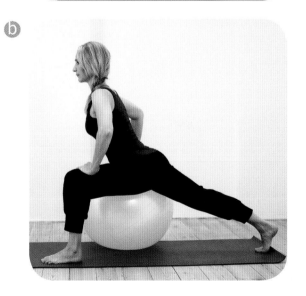

HIP AND BOTTOM STRETCH

? WHAT FOR? To stretch the hip rotators and the bottom.

1 Start seated on the ball with your feet hip width apart.

2 Ⓑ Walk your feet out, allowing the ball to roll up your spine. Stop when the ball is underneath your lower back.

3 Ⓒ Cross your right ankle over your left knee and then drop your hips towards the floor increasing the stretch as far as you can.

4 Hold for up to 20 seconds. Reverse the process to come out of the position. Repeat on the other side.

TIP

- The further you drop your hips towards the floor, the more intense the stretch will be. Adjust your position so that it is comfortable for your body.

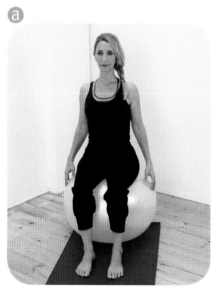

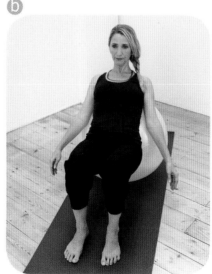

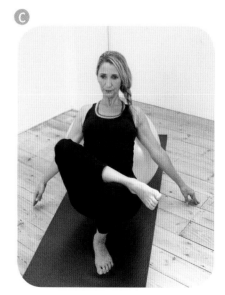

KNEELING INNER THIGH STRETCH

? WHAT FOR? This is a fantastic inner thigh stretch aided by the rolling capabilities of the ball.

1 **a** Start kneeling up with the ball by your right side.

2 **b** Place your left hand on the floor in front of you and the ball underneath your right knee. Once the ball is in position, place your right hand on the floor as well.

3 Roll the ball away from your body and push your hips towards the floor as far as is comfortable. You can hold this stretch for 30–60 seconds. Repeat on the other side.

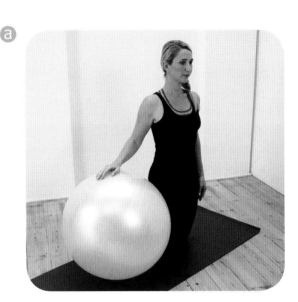

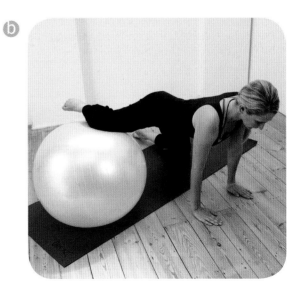

TIPS

- Ensure that you roll the ball away from you in a smooth motion. Don't be tempted to bounce in this stretch as this may lead to pulling a muscle.
- If you would like to increase the intensity of the stretch, try placing the ball underneath your ankle rather than your knee and then rolling the ball away from you as before.

FRONT LYING QUAD STRETCH

? WHAT FOR? To stretch the muscles in the front of the thigh.

1 **(a)** Start on your hands and knees over the ball.

2 **(b)** Walk your weight forwards slightly so that the ball is resting underneath your hips and your weight is equal between your hands and the balls of your feet.

3 **(c)** Now take hold of your right foot with your right hand. Bring your knees together and push your hips towards the ball.

4 Hold this stretch for up to 20 seconds. Repeat on the other leg.

TIPS

- You should feel this stretch down the front of your thigh. If you can't, try moving your weight forwards slightly on the ball and pushing your hips into the ball.
- If you struggle to reach your foot with your hand you can use a towel to give yourself an arm extension! Take a small towel and make a loop out of it with both ends held in your hand. Put your foot into the loop and then pull your foot towards your bottom in the same way as before.

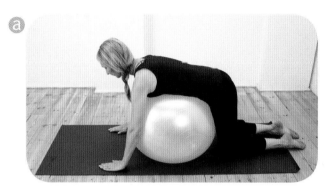

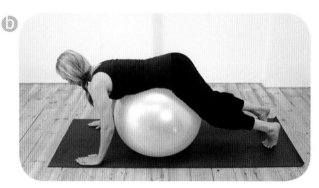

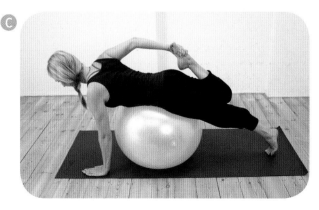

FROG STRETCH

? WHAT FOR? To stretch and increase flexibility of the inner thigh muscles.

1 **ⓐ** Start lying on your back with your arms out to the side or by your sides and feet resting on the ball, soles of your feet together and your knees falling out to the sides.

2 **ⓑ** Roll the ball in, bringing your heels in towards your bottom as much as possible. Now place your hands onto your knees and try and ease them further out, increasing the stretch. Hold for up to a minute or as long as you like!

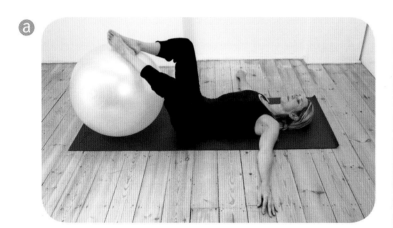

TIP

- This is actually a really nice stretch to just get into and relax for a while. The weight of the knees will gradually increase the stretch as the muscles relax and the rest of the body can just melt into the floor.

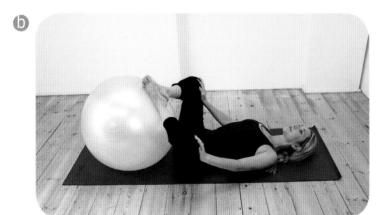

SEATED INNER THIGH STRETCH

? **WHAT FOR?** This is a more intense stretch for the inner thigh muscles. This stretch works perfectly with the ball, as it enables you to gently roll yourself in and out.

1 **a** Start seated on the floor with your legs straight and opened wide and the ball placed in the middle with your hands resting on top.

2 **b** Keeping your legs straight, roll the ball away from you as far as is comfortable and relax your upper body over, bringing your head towards the floor.

3 Hold this stretch for between 30–60 seconds and then roll yourself back in.

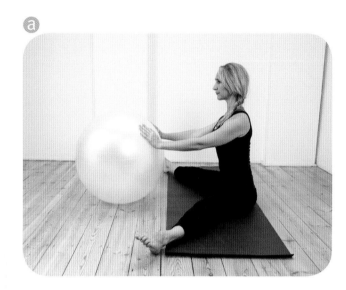

TIPS

- Keep your knees pointing up to the ceiling as you roll forwards. Avoid allowing the knees to roll inwards.
- Get yourself into the stretch, and after 15–20 seconds try to roll a little further forwards, increasing the stretch further.

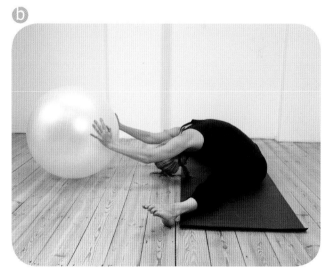

LYING HAMSTRING STRETCH

? WHAT FOR? To stretch and increase the flexibility of the hamstrings.

1 **a** Start lying on your back with your knees bent up, feet flat on the floor and the ball resting on your tummy.

2 **b** Place the ball on your left knee, and then bring your right leg in front of the ball, keeping it extended.

3 Hold the stretch for between 30–60 seconds gradually increasing it if you feel able. Repeat on the other side.

a

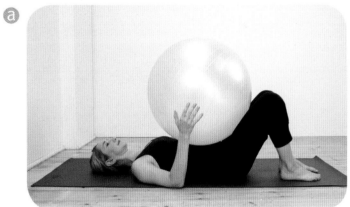

b

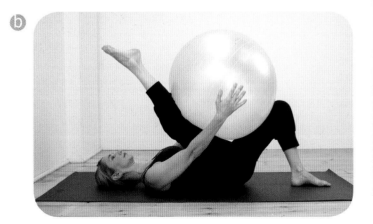

TIP

- To increase the stretch, adjust the position of the ball by moving it further down your supporting leg. You can also use your hands if necessary, to pull the ball further in towards your body.

FULL BODY STRETCHES

BALL SPINE CURLS

? WHAT FOR? This stretch targets the backs of the legs as well as increasing flexibility through the spine and the lower back. It is also about letting go and giving the whole body over to the stretch. The ball really helps you to visualise the rolling of the spine.

1 **ⓐ** Start standing with your feet hip width apart, hugging the ball just underneath your breastbone.

2 **ⓑ** Starting with your head, curl down through your spine allowing the ball to roll down your body and your spine to follow. Keep going until you are as far as you can comfortably go.

3 Hold the stretch for 30–60 seconds and then slowly roll back up to your starting position with the ball leading the way.

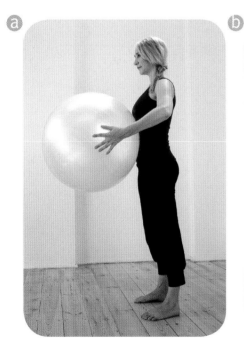
ⓐ

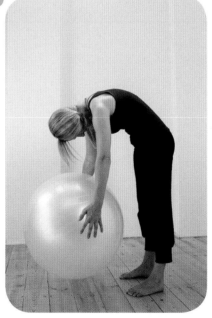
ⓑ

TIP

- Imaging working through each vertebra as you curl though the spine. Hug the ball close; slow down over any areas that feel stiff or tense.

BALL HUG

? WHAT FOR? To stretch the muscles of the upper back and lengthen the spine.

1 ⓐ Start on your hands and knees over the ball, then come down onto your elbows, clasping your hands together.

2 ⓑ Bring your elbows in as close to the ball as possible and relax your head over, feeling a stretch in the spine and upper back.

3 Hold the stretch for up to a minute, or for as long as you feel comfortable.

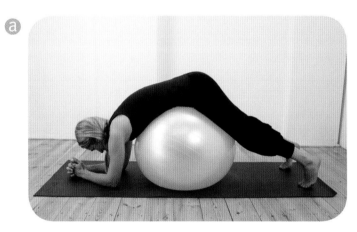

TIP

- Roll yourself around on the ball a little to find a position where you feel you get the best stretch for your body. This is a lovely position you can play around with to suit.

SIDE LYING SIDE STRETCH

? **WHAT FOR?** This gives a lovely stretch all the way up the side of the body. Really enjoy draping yourself over the ball here.

1 Start kneeling up with the ball by your right side.

2 Reach your right arm over the ball resting it onto the floor. Extend your legs into a scissor position with your left leg forwards of your right.

3 Extend both arms over your head so that you are extending right through your body from hands to feet.

4 Hold the stretch for up to a minute, or for as long as you feel comfortable.

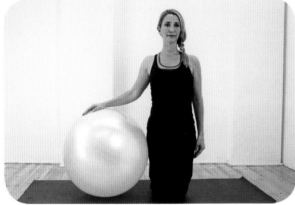

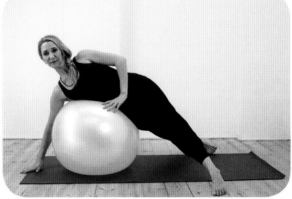

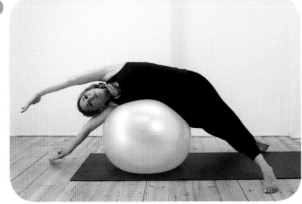

TIPS

• Try to keep your hips and shoulders square on to the front throughout the stretch.
• Imagine you are being pulled in opposite directions from your hands to your feet, so you are fully lengthened through the body.

FULL BODY STRETCH

? WHAT FOR? This is the most wonderful stretch, only made possible by the round nature of the ball. Go into it gently until you gain confidence as it does also require some balancing skills!

1. **a** Start seated on the ball with your feet hip width apart.

2. **b** Walk your feet out, allowing the ball to roll up your spine. Stop when the ball is underneath your lower back.

3. **c** Drop your hips down towards the floor and rest your head back onto the ball.

4. **d** Now extend your legs, pushing yourself backwards until your body is fully draped over the ball.

5. **e** If you feel able, reach your arms over your head.

6. Hold this stretch up to a minute, or for as long as you feel comfortable.

TIP

- Think of lengthening right through the body from fingers to toes. Allow yourself to fully relax in this position and let all of your tension seep away.

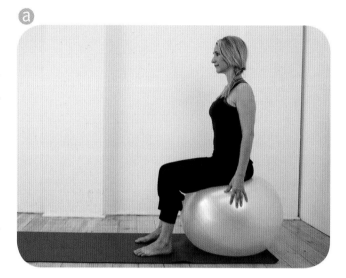

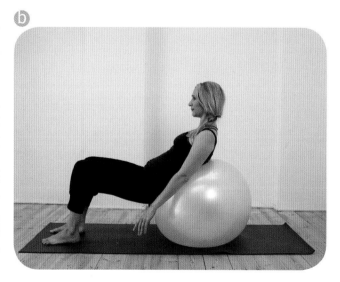

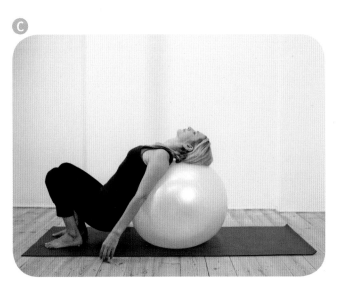

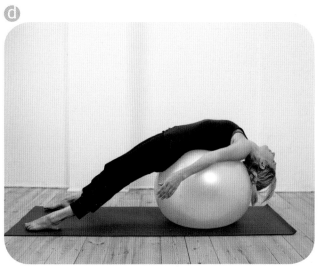

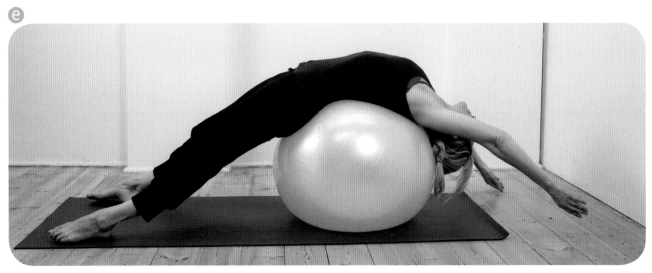

CHAPTER SEVEN

HEALTHY BACK AND POSTURE

INTRODUCTION

'Don't slouch! Sit up straight!' You probably remember being constantly told this during your teenage years. Interestingly when we first start walking, we have naturally good posture; we know how to correctly bend down, pick up objects and stand up straight. Toddlers never slouch. Bad posture is a bad habit, inflicted upon ourselves because of our lifestyle choices.

Alarming and increasing numbers of adults suffer from recurring back and neck pain due to unnecessary stress placed on the spine by bad posture or rounded shoulders, projecting a poor body image and causing low self-esteem.

Posture is the position in which we hold ourselves when we stand, sit or lie. Good posture is the position where the least amount of stress is placed on the spine and supporting joints and ligaments during weight-bearing activity. If we don't practise good posture, over time abnormal stress can lead to structural changes in the spine, including degeneration of disks and joints, lengthening or shortening of the supportive ligaments and muscles, and wear and tear of cartilage. All of these structural changes can lead to pain and other problems, such as chronic headaches and shoulder issues.

Luckily we can all improve our posture quite easily, though if you have spent years standing incorrectly then there will be a bit of re-learning to do. Having good posture not only helps to avoid back and neck pain, it can make you look slimmer, more attractive and it is a real reflection to the outside world of how we see ourselves. In addition it improves breathing and circulation, which can result in less cellulite as well as better overall functioning of the body.

In this chapter we are going to look at strengthening the back and mobilising the spine, particularly working on weak and stiff areas. We are going to open up your posture to try and counteract the amount of time spent leaning forwards hunched over computers, paperwork and driving cars.

If you are a back pain sufferer, be careful with exercises that rotate or extend the spine as these can aggravate an existing condition. Gradually build up strength over time; just listen to your body and do what feels comfortable.

BENEFITS OF GOOD POSTURE

- Keeps bones and joints in proper alignment, ensuring muscles are used correctly.
- Helps to prevent back and muscular pain.
- Helps decrease the abnormal wearing of joint surfaces that could result in arthritis.
- Decreases the stress on the ligaments holding the joints of the spine together.
- Prevents muscles fatigue, as muscles will be used more efficiently.
- Improves breathing.
- Improves circulation.
- Increases energy and helps the body to work more efficiently.
- Contributes to a good appearance.
- Improves body confidence and self-esteem.

CORRECT POSTURE

STANDING

1 Stand with your feet hip width apart, your knees slightly relaxed so that you are not locking the knee joints backwards.

2 Maintain the small natural curve in the lower back, but avoid overarching. Your tail bone should be slightly tucked down. A gentle engagement of the abdominal muscles will keep your spine aligned.

3 Lift from your breastbone, creating space between your ribcage and hips. This will automatically move your shoulder blades down your back.

4 Level your chin so your head tilts neither up nor down.

5 Centre your weight by rocking forwards onto your toes, and then back onto the heels, gradually making the movement smaller and smaller, until you stop in the place where you feel most centred and balanced.

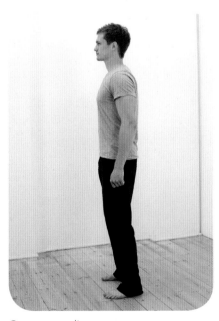

Correct standing posture

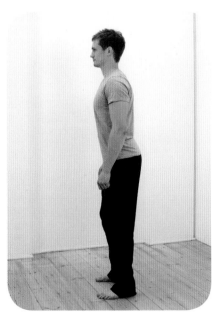

Bad posture 1

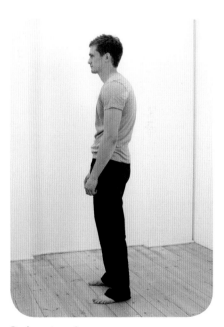

Bad posture 2

SITTING

When seated on a ball you are actively sitting as you have to keep some muscles in action to aid balance and avoid falling off. This has been proven to assist concentration levels and also makes slouching much more difficult than when seated on a chair. Try swapping your office chair for your ball next time you are seated at your computer.

1 Start sitting on your ball with your back straight and your shoulders back.

2 Your feet should be hip width apart and flat on the floor. Make sure your weight is evenly distributed between both hips and feet. Your hips should be level with your knees or slightly higher.

5 When seated, the natural curves in your lower back, upper back and neck should all be present, but be careful not to overarch the lower spine.

6 To help you find neutral spine position, tilt your pelvis forwards and then backwards gradually making the movement smaller and smaller until you come to a halt in the centre.

7 Activate a gentle engagement of the abdominal muscles to cement the position of the spine.

8 Try to avoid sitting in the same position without a break for longer than 30 minutes.

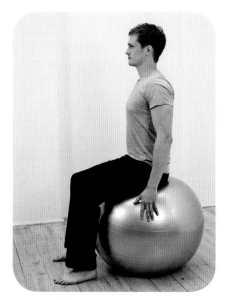

Correct sitting posture

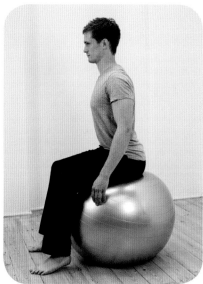

Bad posture 1

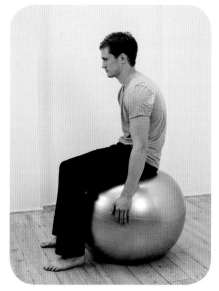

Bad posture 2

LYING

1 When lying down, the spine is most comfortable when neutral position is maintained. The best way to achieve this is to lie on your back, or on your side with your knees slightly bent.

2 Avoid having a mattress that is too soft and avoid sleeping on your stomach, especially if you already have back pain.

3 Your pillow should be placed under your head only – not your shoulders.

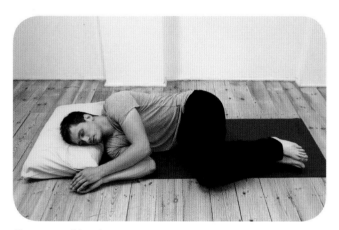

Correct position 1

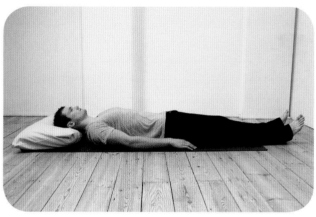

Correct position 2

STRENGTHENING

The following exercises work the muscles in the back to ensure any weak areas are strengthened or maintained. Some focus on core strength, which is essential for supporting the spine. A strong back and core equals a healthy back and good posture.

BACK EXTENSIONS ON THE BALL

? WHAT FOR? To strengthen muscles in the lower back. If you have any underlying back problems or pain you should start very gently with this exercise, or avoid altogether if it aggravates your current problem.

1 **a** Start on your hands and knees over the ball then place your hands lightly on the ball.

2 **b** Keeping the head in line with the rest of your spine, raise your upper body away from the ball.

3 Then relax the body back down. Repeat the extensions 8–12 times.

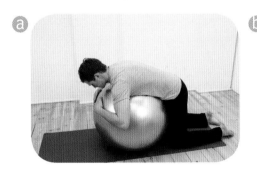

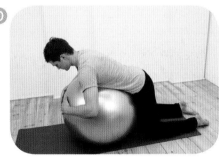

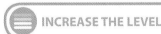
INCREASE THE LEVEL

1 Repeat step 1 as before.
2 Now adjust your weight so that your legs are straight. To increase the level further, place your hands behind your back. **c**
3 Repeat steps 2 and 3 as before.

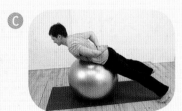

TIPS

- If you have your hands placed on the ball, make sure they are in light contact and only use them to aid your lifting away from the ball.
- Keep your core muscles activated to ensure you don't overarch the spine.
- If necessary, you can perform this exercise with your feet against a wall to aid balance.

LYING BACK EXTENSIONS

? **WHAT FOR?** This exercise is similar to the last and exercises the lower back in the same way. The position is more of a challenge though and you also have the added weight of the ball.

1 **a** Start lying on your front with the ball placed on your upper back and held in place with your hands.

2 **b** Keeping your head in line with the rest of the spine, lift your upper body a few inches away from the floor.

3 Relax back down to your starting position.

4 Repeat the extensions 8–12 times.

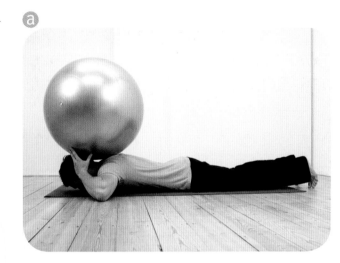

TIPS

- Only lift as far away from the floor as is comfortable.
- Keep the spine extended and core muscles contracted to avoid overarching the lower back.
- Keep your focus down to the floor to ensure your head stays in line with the rest of the spine.
- Try to keep the muscles in your legs and bottom relaxed throughout to ensure the work is coming from the back.

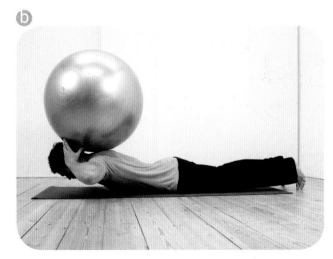

OPPOSITE ARM AND LEG RAISES

? WHAT FOR? To tone the arms, torso and backs of the legs. This exercise is also to practise lengthening through the whole body and learning to centre the weight. This is a follow on from the kneeling version described on page 146.

1 **a** Start on your hands and knees over the ball, and then adjust your weight so that the ball is resting underneath your hips and your weight is equal between your hands and feet.

2 **b** Extend your right arm and left leg away from you along the floor. When you have lengthened as far as possible, allow them to rise off the floor until they are parallel with it.

3 Keep the length through the body as you lower the arm and leg back to your starting position.

4 Repeat on the other side and then 6–8 times, alternating sides.

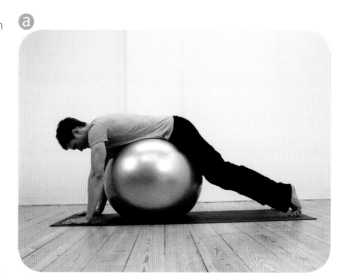

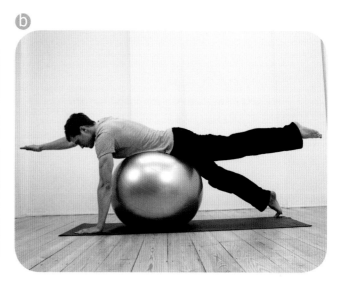

TIPS

- Try to keep your weight centred in your pelvis throughout the exercise. You should not feel a shift from side to side as you change legs.
- Lengthen the arm and leg out only to a neutral position to avoid arching the lower back. Keep your core contraction in place to help maintain the position of the spine.

BRIDGE BALANCE

? WHAT FOR? To strengthen core muscles, challenge stability and encourage a lengthening of the spine.

1 **a** Start lying on your back with your feet resting up on the ball and your arms relaxed down by your sides.

2 **b** Slowly lift your pelvis away from the floor, curling through each vertebra until you are in a straight diagonal line from your shoulders to your feet. Try to keep your shoulder blades back and your chest lifted throughout.

3 **c** Holding the body in this position, reach your arms up towards the ceiling.

4 **d** Now slowly lower your arms over to the right side, keeping balanced, then back to the centre and over to the left.

5 Repeat the arm movement, right and left, 4–6 times, then slowly curl back down to your starting position.

TIPS

- Use your core contraction to lock the spine in the diagonal position. This will aid your balance.
- Keep focused on a fixed point ahead of you to help concentration and balance.

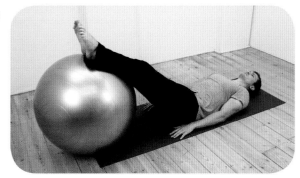

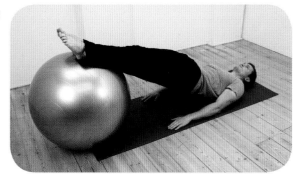

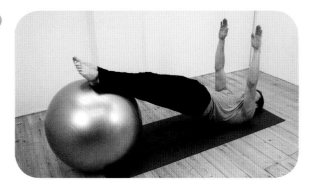

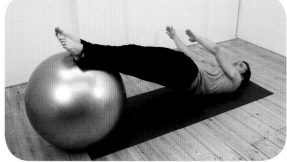

LAT PULL DOWNS AGAINST WALL

For this exercise you will need to find a clear wall wide enough to accommodate the width of the ball.

? WHAT FOR? To tone and strengthen the back. This is also great for opening out the chest and shoulders.

1 Start standing sideways on to the wall, with the ball placed between your forearm and the wall, your arm held at a right angle to your body.

2 **b** Push against the ball to create resistance, roll it down until your elbow is level with your waist.

3 Now roll it back up to your starting position

4 Repeat the rolls 8–12 times. Repeat on the other side.

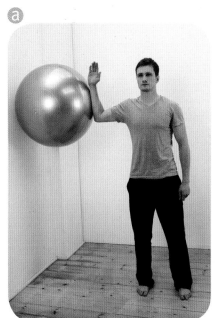

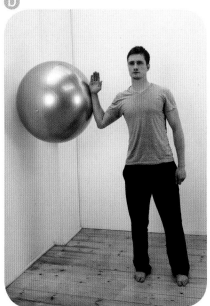

TIPS

- Think about squeezing the shoulder blades together as you roll the ball down to really engage the muscles in the back.
- Keep the shoulder stabilised throughout the exercise.
- Try to minimise any movement elsewhere in the body.

SEATED BALL BALANCE

? WHAT FOR? This is a great exercise for challenging the lengthening of the spine and a centring of your weight. It will strengthen the core and aid balance.

1 **(a)** Start seated on your ball with your feet hip width apart and your hands lightly resting on the ball.

2 **(b)** Try to take your feet off the floor while keeping the spine lengthened.

3 Balance here for as long as you can.

4 **(c)** If you want to, try taking your hands off the ball and reaching your arms out to the sides while balancing.

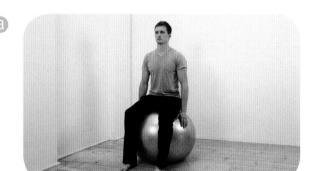

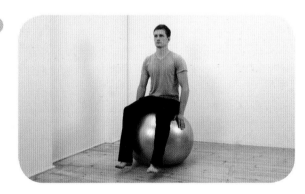

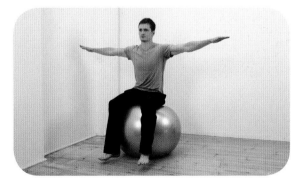

TIPS

- Focus on a fixed point at eye level to help to stay balanced.
- Use your hands on the ball to help you balance initially, until you feel confident enough to take them off.
- Lengthen long through the crown of the head, imagine you have a piece of string pulling you up towards the ceiling.
- Contract your core muscles as this will aid balance as well as maintain your length through the spine.

MOBILITY

The following exercises have an emphasis on maintaining and increasing the mobility of the spine. Listen to your body and allow yourself to really work through areas that feel particularly stiff or tight, perhaps slowing down the movement at these points to give them a little extra attention.

SEATED CURL DOWNS

? WHAT FOR? To mobilise the spine and find your centre of gravity on the ball. A great exercise for loosening up any tense spots in the spine.

1 **a** Start seated on the ball with your feet hip width apart and your arms relaxed by your sides.

2 **b** Starting from your head, curl down slowly through the spine as far as your flexibility will allow.

3 Once at the bottom of the movement, start curling back up to your starting position, making sure your head arrives last.

4 Repeat the curl downs 4–6 times

TIPS

- The head leads the movement on the way down and then is the last body part to arrive on the way up.
- Make sure you work through each vertebra as you curl down through the spine. On the way back up, visualise stacking the vertebrae one on top of the other as you come up to sitting.
- Take this exercise slowly and really use it as an opportunity to massage through the spine, slowing down even more through any spots that feel stiff or tense.
- Keep your arms relaxed throughout the movement.

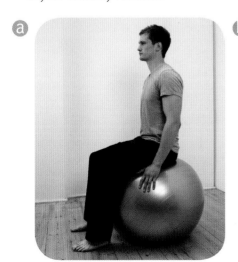
a

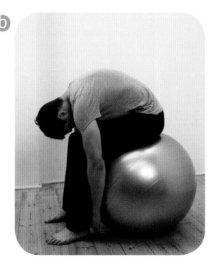
b

ROTATING CURLS

? WHAT FOR? To rotate and mobilise the spine. Great for emphasising neutral spine position each time you return.

1 **a** Start seated on the ball with your feet hip width apart and your arms extended out to the sides.

2 **b** Rotate from your waist around to the right side, keeping your hips square on to the front.

3 **c** Keeping the rotation in place, curl down as far as your flexibility will allow. Let the arms relax down.

4 **d** Curl back up returning to your rotated position and bring your arms back out to the sides.

5 Now rotate back until you are facing forwards in your starting position.

6 Repeat on the other side, then alternate sides for 4–6 repetitions.

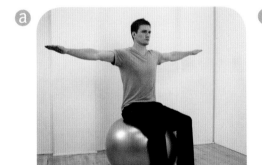

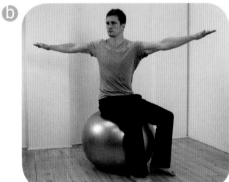

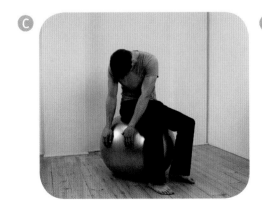

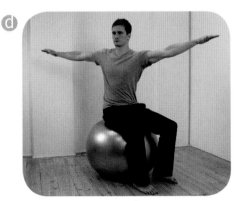

TIPS

- Engage your core muscles before starting this exercise to ensure you don't over-rotate the spine.
- Try to complete the whole exercise in a flowing motion without stops and starts, keeping the same speed throughout.

CHEST LIFTS

? WHAT FOR? To increase flexibility and strength in the upper back. This is also a lovely exercise to open out across the chest.

1 **a** Start standing with your feet hip width apart and the ball lifted up, as if you are reaching towards the opposite edge of the ceiling.

2 **b** Keeping the ball still, lift your head and chest towards the ceiling. Be careful not to arch from your lower back.

3 Hold the position for about 10 seconds then relax. Repeat the lifts six times.

TIPS

- Engage your core muscles before starting the exercise. This will stabilise the lower spine and ensure that the movement comes from the upper back.
- Imagine that you have a piece of string attached to the centre of your breast bone, and you are being lifted from this point.
- When you return to the centre at the end of the exercise try to keep with you the feeling of openness through the chest that you have created.

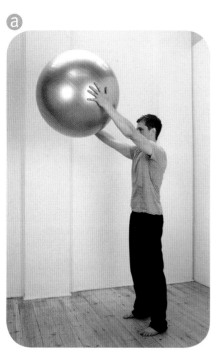

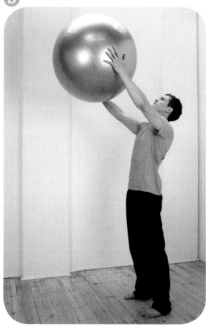

BALL REACHES

? WHAT FOR? This exercise practises extending and curling through the spine. It will increase strength in the lower back as well as mobility throughout the spine. It is also good practice for correct lifting techniques – see the body mechanics section on page 236.

1 Start standing with your feet hip width apart and the ball reaching up above your head.

2 **b** Engage your core muscles to start, then keeping an extended spine and your arms above your head, bend from your hips lowering your torso down until the ball is reaching towards the floor. Go as far as your flexibility will allow while keeping a flat back.

3 **c** When you are at your lowest position, relax the spine and then curl back up to standing, coming up through one vertebra at a time.

4 Repeat 4–6 times.

TIPS

- When lowering the body in the flat back position, try to keep a straight line from the ball through your shoulders and to your hips.
- Only lower down in your flat back position as far as you can maintain a straight spine. Once you have gone as far as you can in this position, relax the spine allowing it to curve, then start to curl back up to standing.
- If necessary you can bend your knees slightly throughout the exercise to allow you a greater range of movement.

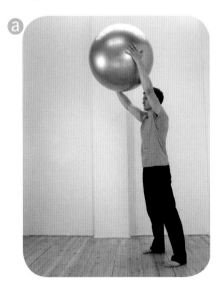

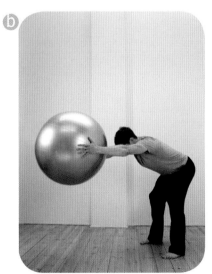

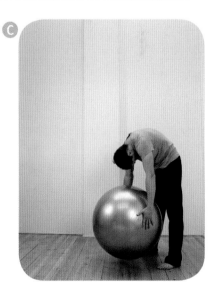

CHEST OPENINGS

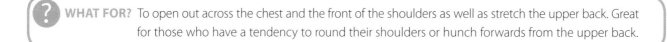

? **WHAT FOR?** To open out across the chest and the front of the shoulders as well as stretch the upper back. Great for those who have a tendency to round their shoulders or hunch forwards from the upper back.

1 **a** Start on your hands and knees over the ball. Walk yourself forwards so that the ball is underneath your hips and your weight is evenly distributed between your hands and feet.

2 **b** Thread your right hand underneath your left arm, reaching as far as you can until you feel a stretch across your upper back.

3 **c** Now bring the right arm back out and keep reaching it all the way up to the ceiling, then back as far as you can behind you. Keep both hips in contact with the ball here.

4 Repeat steps 2 and 3 4–6 times. Then repeat on the other side.

TIPS

- Keep both hips firmly on the ball throughout the exercise.
- You should feel a stretch in the upper back when reaching under and a stretch across the chest when opening up.

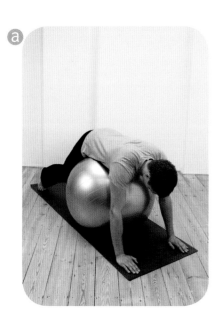

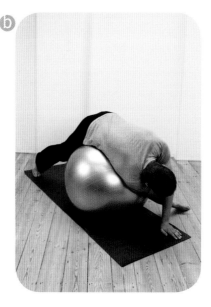

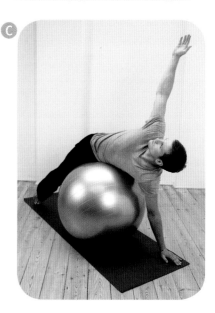

CHEST STRETCH

? WHAT FOR? To stretch and open up through the chest and shoulders. Great for reversing a 'hunched' posture.

1 **ⓐ** Start kneeling up with the ball placed on the floor behind you. Gently lean yourself back on the ball so that it is resting just underneath your shoulder blades.

2 **ⓑ** Reach your arms back as far as you can and lift your chest and face towards the ceiling until you can feel a stretch across your chest and shoulders.

3 Hold the stretch for as long as you are comfortable and then relax.

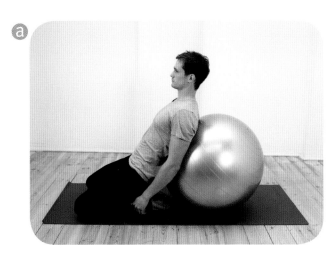

TIP

- The great thing about having a ball here is you arch yourself around it, enabling you to mould your chest into an open position. Try to keep hold of this feeling once you come off the ball.

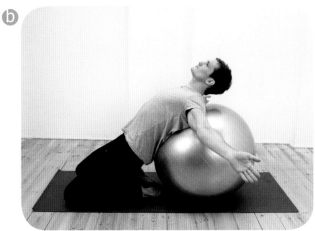

GOOD BODY MECHANICS

Good body mechanics is the way you position your body when going about your everyday jobs. Learning how to use good body mechanics in everyday life is very important if you want to avoid, or manage, back and neck pain and improve posture.

Whenever your body is out of neutral alignment you are automatically putting excess strain on your back, but keeping a good alignment and using good body mechanics in your daily routines can help to eliminate unnecessary problems. Working on an exercise ball is already holding you in good stead, as functional fitness is one of its great strengths. You can also use your ball to help you practise for the following situations.

STANDING JOBS

- Always try and stand close to the job that you are doing. For example if it is ironing, stand close to the board rather than having to lean forwards.
- If you are standing in one place for a long time, try altering your position by putting one knee or foot up on something – your ball works really well here.

LIFTING

- Try not to lift anything alone if it is too heavy (more than half your body weight would be a good measure).
- When picking up an object, bend from your knees and keep your back straight. It is when you bend from the waist that you put your spine under unnecessary strain.
- Make sure you are close to the object that you want to lift, rather than leaning out to reach for it.

- Before you pick the object up, engage your core muscles.
- Once you are holding the object, keep it close to your centre of gravity (your navel).
- Avoid twisting from the waist while holding the object; turn by moving your feet instead.
- Try not to lift an object above waist level as this will increase the pressure on the lower back.
- Practise lifting with your ball. This is a great way to master your technique while strengthening the working muscles.

SITTING AT A COMPUTER

- When seated make sure you can place your feet flat on the floor, and your knees and hips are at the same height. If not you will need to lower your chair or use a footrest. You can also use your ball to sit on, adjusting the amount of air in it to achieve the correct height.
- You should sit up tall with your core muscles activated.
- Have your computer screen at the correct height and directly in front of you so that you do not need to look up, down or to one side.
- Try not to remain in one position for too long. Get up, stretch and move around whenever possible.
- Use your ball chair to double up as something to stretch over in one of your breaks.

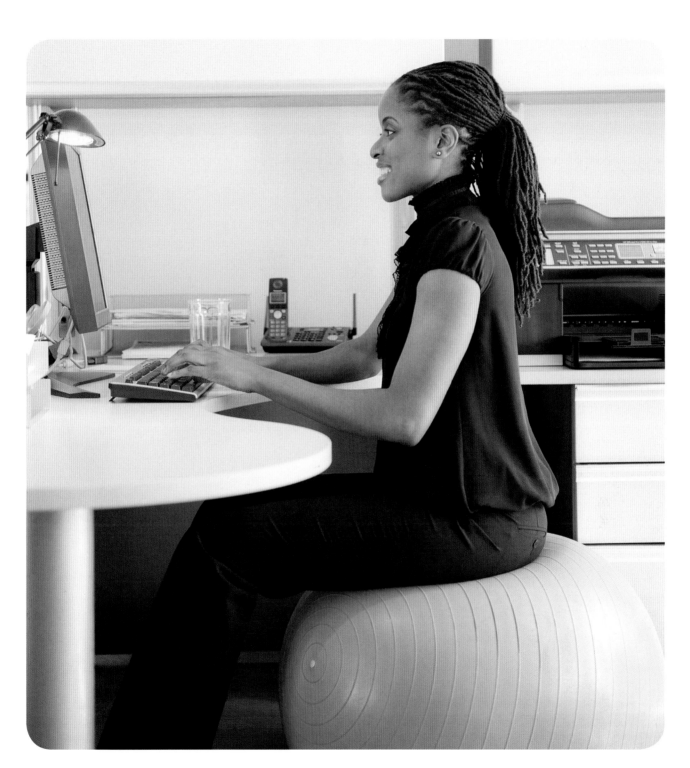

CHAPTER EIGHT

PREGNANCY, BIRTHING AND BEYOND

INTRODUCTION

My son will be four years old in a couple of weeks and yet it seems like only yesterday that I sat on my ball doing antenatal exercises, amazed at how even during pregnancy the ball had so much to offer. I was already a convert, but a lot of people have their first introduction to the ball during their pregnancy and go on to use it through birth and as a postnatal exercise tool to help regain their pre-pregnancy shape.

During pregnancy, exercise is not about increasing your fitness level, but about maintaining current levels with an ever-challenging body shape and size.

Throughout pregnancy the ball can offer postural relief alongside a challenging workout. It offers a way to position the body during exercise that is safe for mother and baby as well as an opportunity to practise birthing positions, such as: squatting with support from the ball (rather than needing a partner), strengthening the muscles needed for a more active birth, opening up the pelvis ready for the big day. The ball provides a firm yet soft place to sit, forcing good posture and reducing the chance of muscle strain. It keeps the supportive muscles of the spine in shape and offers an alternative to sitting in a chair, which becomes increasingly uncomfortable during the last trimester. Sitting on your ball in your last few weeks of pregnancy will also help the baby move into the right position for birth, potentially reducing labour time.

During labour more and more women and midwives are beginning to realise the benefits of a more active birth.

This allows you the freedom to move around during labour rather than lying in one position on your back. It has been proven to reduce labour time, the chance of an assisted delivery, tearing and abnormal foetal heart-rate problems. The ball, known as a 'birthing ball' in this environment, can play a vital role in offering an alternative to being on a bed. It offers the woman a choice of positions in which she can keep the pelvis mobile and open, giving her the freedom to change positions to help manage the pain through contractions. Moving around during labour helps increase blood flow to the placenta, and prevents foetal distress.

After the birth, the ball is a fantastic tool that will help you regain your pre-pregnancy shape in no time at all. You can start exercising your pelvic floor muscles straight away, although you will need to wait until after your six-week check to embark on a full exercise routine (even longer if you were delivered through a Caesarian section). We will also be looking at exercises you can do with your baby as well as during those few rare moments when you find yourself alone.

BENEFITS OF EXERCISING DURING PREGNANCY

- Increased mental and physical well-being
- Reduced risk of gestational diabetes
- Reduced risk of induced hypertension
- Reduction in labour time
- Increased chance of natural birth – no intervention
- Less risk of loss of bladder control during and after pregnancy
- More chance of a quick return to pre-pregnancy figure

SAFETY POINTS

- Always consult with your doctor or midwife before commencing any exercise programme during pregnancy.
- In pregnancy your centre of gravity changes, making balancing a little more challenging. Try using a slightly larger ball that's a little less inflated to give you a more stable base of support.
- As pregnancy progresses, the hormone relaxin will increase in your body, softening your connective tissues in preparation for the birth. This means you need to be extra careful when stretching and extending joints as the risk of injury is increased. Relaxin can stay in your system for up to 5 months after giving birth.
- After the first trimester it is not advisable to lie flat on your back for longer than 30 seconds.
- Avoid high impact, high intensity exercise and always listen to your body – if it is uncomfortable then stop.

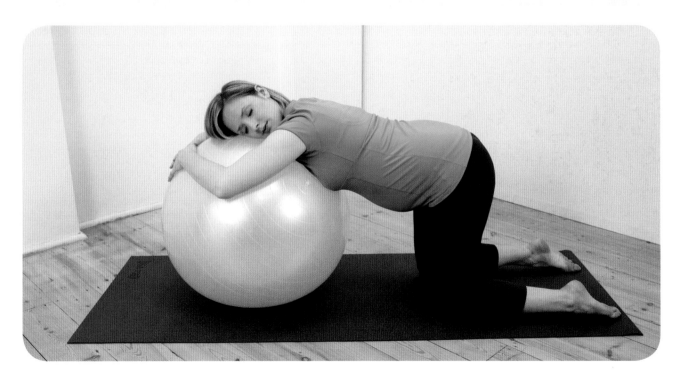

ANTENATAL EXERCISES

SIDE-TO-SIDE BALL ROCKS

? **WHAT FOR?** To open up the pelvis, and strengthen the legs.

1 **a** Start seated at the front of your ball with the legs wide and turned out from the hips. Keep your hands placed on the ball behind you for support.

2 **b** Slowly roll over to the right side, bending the right knee as far as is comfortable.

3 Now slowly roll all the way over to the left side.

4 Keep rolling from side to side for 8–10 repetitions.

TIPS

• Keep your bottom at the front of the ball to get a feeling of opening through the hips and pelvis.
• Keep the movement controlled throughout.

a

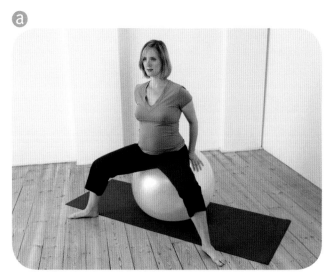

b

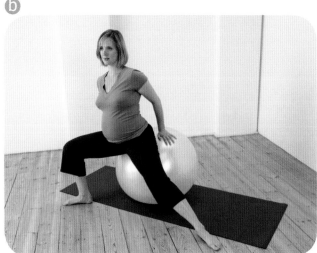

KNEELING CAT STRETCH

? **WHAT FOR?** To release tension from the spine. A great exercise for momentarily taking the pressure off!

1 **ⓐ** Start kneeling with the ball placed on the floor in front of you and your forearms resting against the ball.

2 **ⓑ** Breathe out as you round all the way up the spine and into the neck.

3 Breathe in as you return to a neutral position with the spine.

4 Repeat the Cat Stretch 4–6 times.

TIPS

- Do not arch the back when returning to neutral position as the weight of the baby can add too much pressure to the lower back.
- Keep the movement small if necessary.

ⓐ

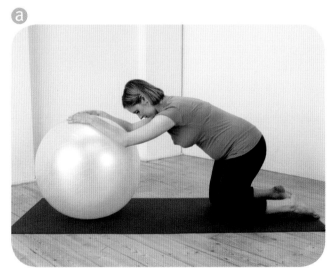

ⓑ

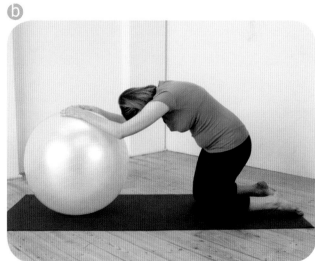

PELVIC CIRCLES

? **WHAT FOR?** To loosen up the hips and release tension from the lower back.

1 Start seated on the ball with your feet hip width apart and your hands lightly touching the sides of the ball for support.

2 **b** Start circling the hips to the right, first pushing them forwards, then to the side, to the back, and then back to the centre.

3 **c** Now take the circle to the left side.

4 Take 4–6 circles, alternating sides.

TIPS

- Keep the movement steady and controlled.
- Avoid making the movement too big. Just as far as is comfortable for you and your baby.

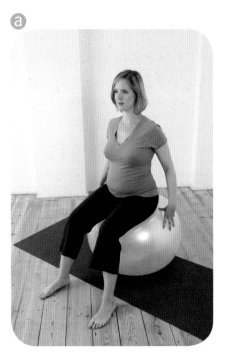

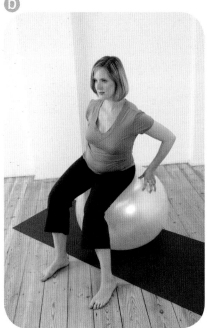

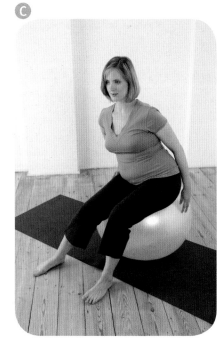

FORWARD BEND WITH WIDE LEGS

? WHAT FOR? To mobilise the spine and open up the hips and pelvis.

1 **ⓐ** Start seated on your ball with your legs wide and turned out from the hips.

2 **ⓑ** Curl down, starting with the head, as far as your bump will allow. Rest your elbows on your knees for support here if necessary, otherwise place your hands on the floor.

3 Hold for a few seconds and then roll back up to your seated position.

4 Take the roll 3–4 times.

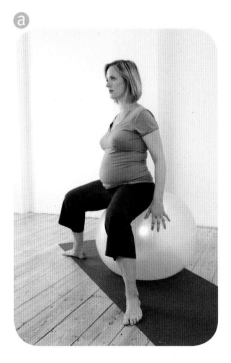

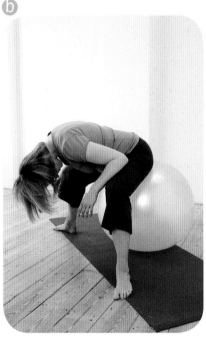

TIPS

- Listen to your body and only do what is comfortable.
- You may find that you need to move yourself to the front of the ball to accommodate your bump while in the forward bend.

PRESS UPS AGAINST THE WALL

? **WHAT FOR?** To tone the muscles in the chest and the back of the arms.

1 Find a clear wall and place your ball on the wall in front of you at chest height. Take a step away from the wall and make sure your feet are hip width apart.

2 **b** Bend your arms, lowering yourself in towards the ball.

3 Straighten your arms again, but don't lock the elbows.

4 Take 6–8 press ups.

TIPS

- If necessary step your feet in closer to the wall and keep the movement small until you gain confidence.
- Keep your core muscles engaged to protect the lower back.
- Keep your hands shoulder width apart on the ball to give you a wide base of support.

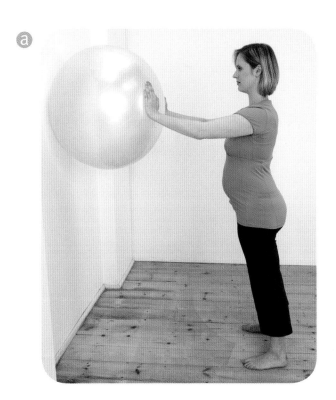

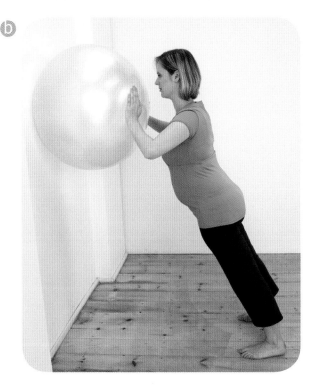

PELVIC FLOOR EXERCISES

 WHAT FOR? It is very important to do some pelvic floor exercises during and after pregnancy, as these muscles can become weakened due to the pressure from the baby and through the birthing process. These muscles play an important role in preventing stress incontinence after birth or further into the future. You don't want to find every time you sneeze or jump that you have a leakage! Toning the pelvic floor muscles is also considered to reduce the risk of tearing the perineum during birth.

1 Start seated on the ball with your feet hip width apart and lean your body forwards slightly so that your elbows are resting onto your knees.

2 Tighten the muscles around your vagina (as if you are trying to stop urine mid-flow), hold for 4–6 seconds, then relax.

3 Repeat up to 20 times. You can also try doing this exercise on other occasions while going about your daily tasks.

TIP

- If you are not sure you are using the right muscles, try this exercise while going to the toilet.

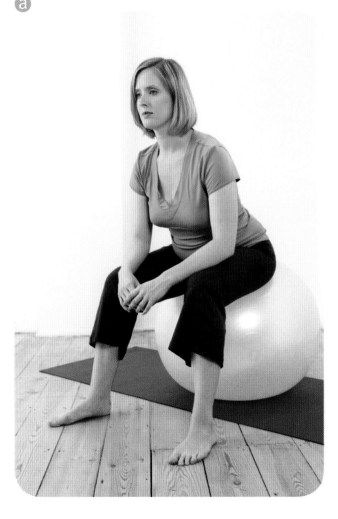

ADDITIONAL ANTENATAL EXERCISES

The following exercises from throughout the book can also be included as part of your antenatal exercise programme. Try including an exercise for each area of the body per session and vary them each time you work out. Remember to avoid doing anything you find uncomfortable.

Chapter 2: Toning & Strengthening   **Ball front raises** (page 54)
Wall squats (page 62)
Ball squats (page 64)
Chest press (page 86) – do not lie flat on your back during this exercise, stay in a 45-degree incline position on the ball
Front raises (page 88)
Bicep curls (page 89)

Chapter 3: Aerobics   **Seated bounces** (page 98)
Step touch (page 99)
Stand up sit downs (page 100)
Jacks (page 102)
Standing arm lifts (page 103)
Lunges with arms (page 104)
Single side steps (page 108)
Double side steps (page 109)
Marching with ball punches (page 110)
Hamstring curls (page 117)
Donkey jumps (page 119)

Chapter 4: Pilates   **Spine twist** (page 133)
Knee lifts with ball rolls (page 134)
Side bend (page 135)
Arm circles (page 137)
Shoulder isolations (page 138)

Chapter 5: Yoga

One leg balance (page 167)
Side bend (page 168)
Forward fold (page 169)
Chair pose (page 170)
Pyramid pose (page 172)
Warrior 1 (page 173)
Warrior 2 (page 174)
Temple pose (page 178)
Tree pose (page 180)
Side plank (page 189)

Chapter 6: Ball Stretches

Standing cat stretch (page 199)
Seated tricep stretch (page 201)
Kneeling chest stretch (page 202)
Lunge stretch (page 206)
Kneeling inner thigh stretch (page 208)
Seated inner thigh stretch (page 211)
Side lying side stretch (page 215)

Chapter 9: De-stress

Seated candle meditation (page 272)
Mind body scan (page 274) – this exercise will need to be modified so that
instead of lying flat on your back you lie at a 45-degree incline position against
something such as a cushion. When you get to the abdominal area try focusing
on your baby for a moment covering it in warmth and love.
Kneeling shoulder massage (page 277)
Upper back/neck massage (page 280)
Buttocks massage (page 281)

BIRTHING WITH THE BALL

These are some positions for you to try while in labour. You may find some work for you and others don't – that's okay. You are also free to experiment with the ball and use it in any way that brings you maximum comfort. This is obviously a very personal experience, do what is right for you.

WIDE LEG SEATED POSITION

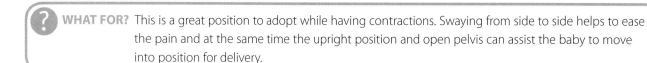

? **WHAT FOR?** This is a great position to adopt while having contractions. Swaying from side to side helps to ease the pain and at the same time the upright position and open pelvis can assist the baby to move into position for delivery.

1 **ⓐ** Start seated on the ball with your legs out wide. Lean forwards, resting your forearms onto your thighs.

2 Gently sway from side to side if you like, or alternatively you can stay still, whichever gives you greatest comfort.

ⓐ

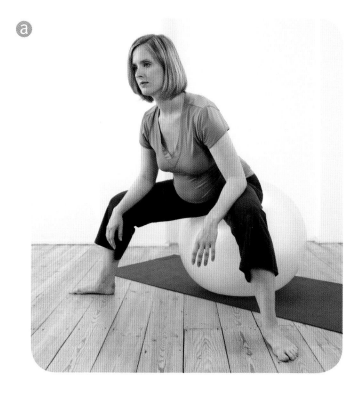

KNEELING FORWARD WITH BALL SUPPORT

? WHAT FOR? This is a great position to ease lower back pain during labour. This position is also useful if your baby is facing forwards and you would like to try and encourage the baby to turn into the optimum birthing position.

1 **a** Start on your knees with the ball in front of you. Drape yourself over the ball so that it is resting under your chest.

2 You can either just relax in this position, or try rocking the pelvis in and out or side to side to ease lower back pain.

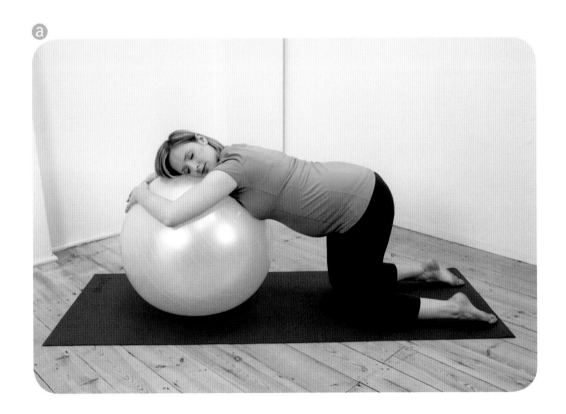

SQUATTING AGAINST THE BALL

? **WHAT FOR?** This position will widen the pelvic outlet ready for birth whilst offering lower back support.

1 **a** Start seated on the ball, then walk your feet forwards, allowing the ball to roll up your spine until it is resting in your lower back.

2 **b** Now bend your knees and drop your hips towards the floor, keeping the feet wider than hip width apart.

3 Try to relax the upper body against the ball. If necessary you can rest the ball against a wall to offer more stability.

a
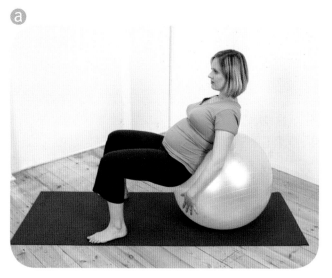

b
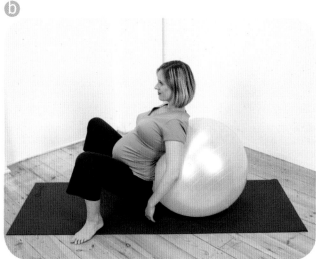

STANDING LEAN

? **WHAT FOR?** A comfortable position that offers pelvic mobility and a resting place for the upper body.

1 **a** Start by placing your ball up on a chair, bed or surface of a similar height.

2 **b** Make sure you are a stride's distance away from the ball and step your feet out to wider than hip width apart. Lean onto the ball, hugging your arms around it and resting your head against it.

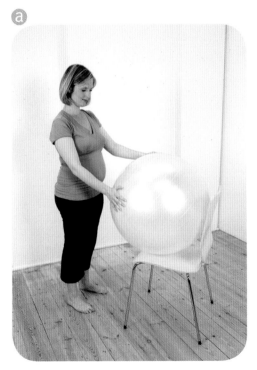

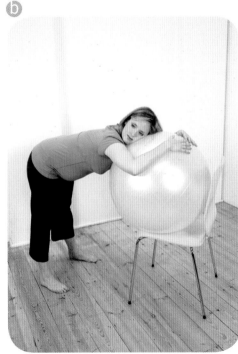

POSTNATAL EXERCISES

PRE SIX-WEEK CHECK

You should abstain from a full exercise programme until after you have been given the all clear at your six-week check. However, there are a few things you can do in the meantime to aid the return to your pre-pregnancy tone and shape. You should try and keep as active as possible; going for lots of walks with your baby is a good way of achieving this, while having the added benefit of getting them off to sleep! The following two exercises are also ideal for you in this period.

CAESAREAN DELIVERY

If you delivered by Caesarean section you will need to wait even longer than 6 weeks before you can start an exercise programme. You will need to avoid any lifting and gradually increase your activity levels as time passes. Gentle walking is a good way of keeping active as soon as you feel up to it and the following pelvic floor exercises are something you too can be getting on with. Take advice from your doctor or midwife as to when you should start doing more.

PELVIC FLOOR

? WHAT FOR? Very similar to the pelvic floor exercise in the antenatal section, these will increase tone in the pelvic muscles after the trauma of the birth, preventing future incontinence problems.

1 Start on your hands and knees over the ball, and then relax your upper body so that your forearms come to the floor, your head rests against your hands and your knees come slightly off the floor.

2 Tighten the muscles around your vagina as if you are trying to stop urine mid-flow. Hold for up to 10 seconds and then relax.

3 Repeat as many times as you like, varying the speed and the amount of time you hold the contraction.

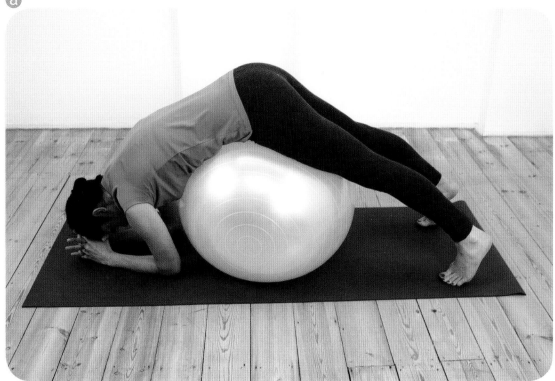

ABDOMINAL BRACING

? WHAT FOR? To start gently toning the abdominal muscles.

1 **ⓐ** Start on your hands and knees over the ball, making sure your spine is in a neutral position and your hands and knees are hip width apart.

2 Try and draw your navel in towards your spine as if you are trying to lift your tummy away from the ball.

3 Hold for up to 10 seconds and repeat 10–15 times.

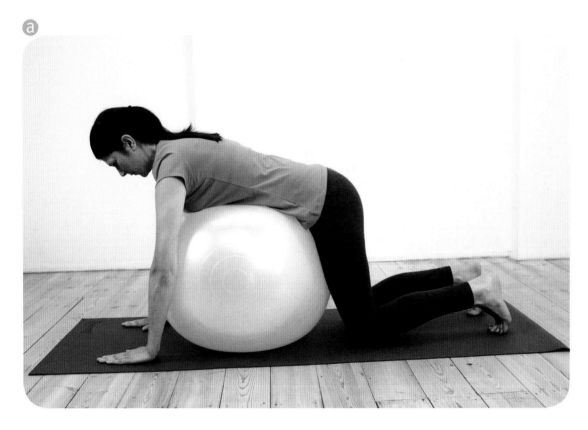

ⓐ

POST SIX-WEEK CHECK

Following your six-week check, if you have been given the all clear by your doctor, you are ready to start exercising gently. You need to listen to your body and gradually increase the level and duration of your routine as and when you feel ready. Finding time to exercise is sometimes one of the biggest challenges during this postnatal stage, so I have included exercises that you can easily do with your baby. Just be aware that some of the exercises will require your baby to have some strength in their neck before you try them. I am sure you and your baby will have lots of fun trying to come up with some more to add to these!

The other exercises in this section have been selected from the rest of the book as a good starting point for you at this stage, but as always, listen to your body and if anything feels uncomfortable don't do it. You should select from these exercises a couple for each body area: upper body, lower body, torso, abdominals. Very quickly you will feel able to add more intense and challenging exercises to your programme; at this point I would advise you to start dipping into the rest of the book again, and gradually increase the level of your workouts over time.

ABDOMINAL SEPARATION

During pregnancy your abdominal muscles separate to make way for the growing baby and it is important that you allow them to close up again before embarking on an abdominal workout. This usually happens fairly quickly, but in some cases can take longer.

Perform the following check to see if you are ready to start some abdominal exercises:

1 Start lying on your back with your knees bent and your feet flat on the floor. Place your little fingers in your belly button and then your other fingers in a row coming towards your ribs.

2 Now lift your head and shoulders slightly off the floor, as if you are performing a small curl and at the same time press down with your fingertips. If you feel a gap, that's the separation know as *diastasis recti*. You will feel the muscles close in around your fingers as you lift. You can try the test again with your little fingers starting slightly below your belly button.

3 Measure how wide the gap is by turning your fingers and measuring the gap in finger widths. You should not start abdominal exercises until the gap is less than two finger widths.

EXERCISES WITH BABY

FORWARD BABY RAISES

 WHAT FOR? To tone and strengthen the muscles in your shoulders and arms.

1 **a** Start seated on your ball with your feet hip width apart and your baby sitting on your legs.

2 **b** Hold your baby around the middle, then keeping your arms extended, lift your baby up in front of you to head height.

3 Now lower your baby back down onto your legs.

4 Repeat the lifts 10–15 times, although this will obviously vary depending on the weight of your baby!

TIPS

- Make sure as you lift your baby that you keep your spine straight and don't allow your weight to tip backwards.
- Keep your core muscles contracted to support your lower back.

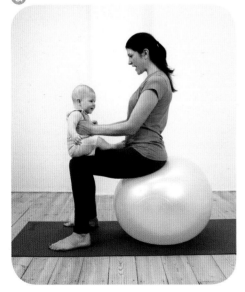

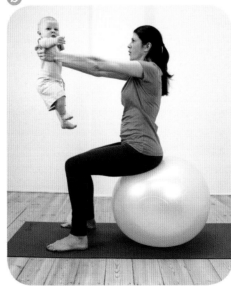

BABY CHEST PRESS

? WHAT FOR? To tone and strengthen the muscles in your chest and the back of your arms.

1 **a** Start lying on the floor on your back with your legs resting up on top of the ball, your knees bent. Lie your baby on their front on your chest holding around their torso.

2 **b** Extend your arms, pushing your baby away from you so that they are level with your chest.

3 Now bend your arms again, coming back to your starting position.

4 Repeat the chest presses 10–15 times.

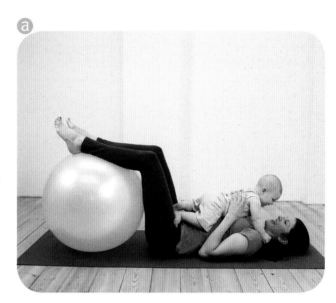

TIPS

- Contract your core muscles to ensure that neutral spine position is maintained throughout the exercise.
- When your arms are in the extended position, keep your elbows slightly soft to avoid locking into the joint.

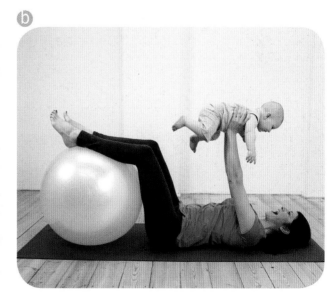

PEEK-A-BOO ROWS

? WHAT FOR? To tone the upper back while entertaining your baby!

1 **a** Start on your hands and knees over the ball with your baby placed on the floor, level with your head. Now cover your face with your hands.

2 **b** Lift your arms, leading with your elbows, as far as you can behind your torso. At the same time you can say 'peek-a-boo' to your baby as you uncover your face!

3 Now return to your starting position.

4 Repeat the rows 10–15 times.

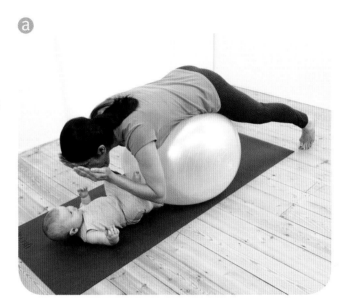

TIPS

- Keep your torso firmly in position as you pull the elbows backwards. There shouldn't be any movement other than from the arms.
- Squeeze your shoulder blades together as the arms pull back to ensure you are really using the muscles in the back.

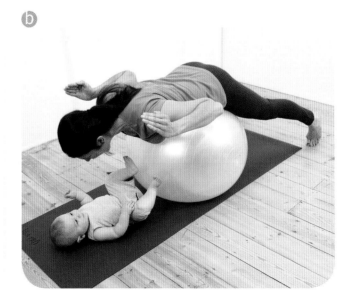

BABY CURL UPS

? **WHAT FOR?** To tone and strengthen the abdominals.

1 **a** Start seated on the ball with your feet hip width apart and your baby sitting on your legs.

2 **b** Now walk out a few steps allowing the ball to roll up your spine until it is underneath your lower back. Adjust your baby so they are sitting on your pelvis.

3 **c** Curl your upper body up as far as is comfortable, then slowly lower back to your starting position.

4 Repeat the curls 10–15 times.

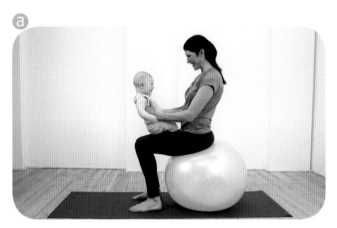

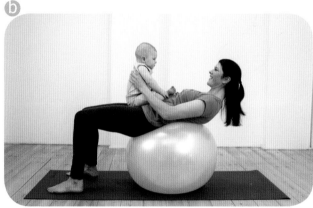

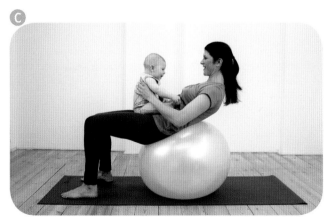

TIPS

- Keep your feet in a wide position to give yourself a good base of support.
- Try and keep your neck in line with the rest of your spine, and avoid any tension here.

ROCK AND SQUAT

? WHAT FOR? To tone and strengthen muscles in the legs and bottom. A lovely comforting position for your baby.

1 **a** Start seated on your ball with your baby rested on your legs. Walk yourself forwards allowing the ball to roll up your spine until it is underneath your lower back.

2 **b** Now bend your knees and drop your hips towards the floor. Hold your baby in close to your chest, facing in towards you, then rest your head back onto the ball.

3 **c** Now straighten your legs a little, rolling backwards over your ball.

4 Bend your knees again, squatting back down to your previous position.

5 Take 10–15 squats and then carefully walk yourself back up onto the ball to finish.

a

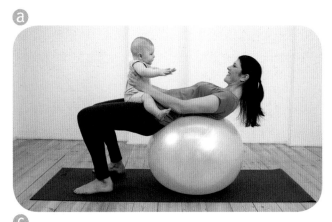

b

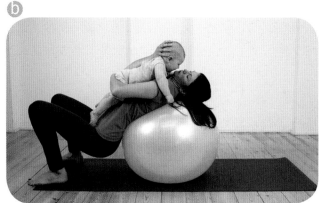

c

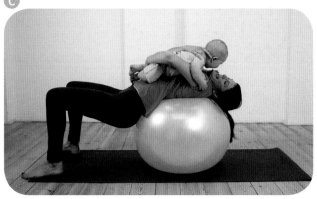

TIPS

- Keep your knees aligned over your ankles while taking your squats
- Keep your body relaxed onto the ball and allow the legs to do all the work.

CALF RAISES

? **WHAT FOR?** To tone the calf muscles, using your baby as a weight.

1 **a** Start seated on your ball with your feet together and your baby lying on your legs.

2 **b** Raise your heels off the floor, pushing up onto the balls of your feet.

3 Now lower the heels back down to your starting position.

4 Repeat the calf raises 20–30 times.

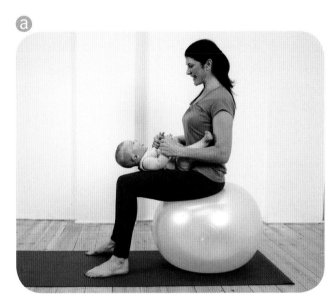

TIP

- Squeeze the calf muscles as you lift the heels to make the muscles work a little bit harder.

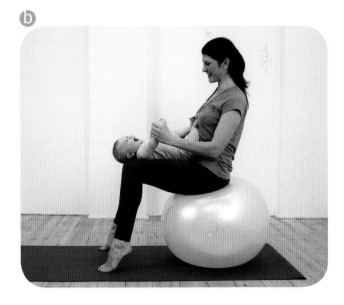

ADDUCTOR SQUEEZES

? **WHAT FOR?** To tone the muscles of the inner thigh.

1 Start sitting on the floor with your feet flat, your knees bent up and the ball held between them. Sit your baby on top of the ball and hold them there.

2 Squeeze your ball with your knees as if you are trying to burst it and then release again.

3 Take 15–20 squeezes.

TIP

- Try to establish a rhythm with your squeezes, so you squeeze, relax, squeeze, relax. You can also try taking some faster pulses as well, anything up to 50!

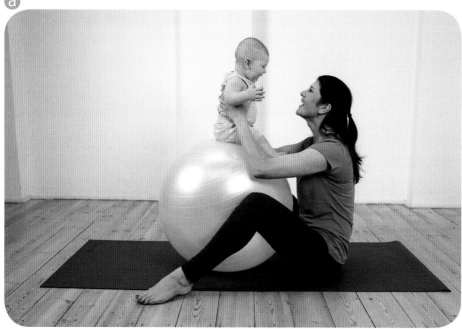

REAR LEG RAISES WITH A RASPBERRY!

? WHAT FOR? To tone and strengthen the backs of the legs and the bottom.

1 **a** Start on your hands and knees over the ball with your baby on the floor in front of you.

2 **b** Take your weight forwards slightly so that your knees come off the floor and your legs are straight. Rest your forearms on the floor either side of your baby.

3 **c** Raise your straight legs up behind you until your body is in a diagonal line, then lower back to your starting position. You can blow a sneaky raspberry on your baby's tummy at the same time as lifting!

4 Repeat the lifts 10–15 times.

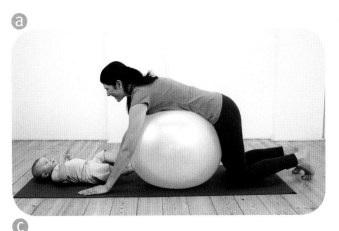
a

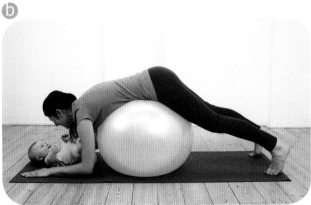
b

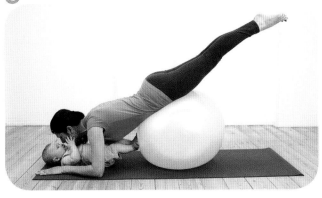
c

TIPS

- Make sure that your core contraction is in place before starting the exercise as this will ensure neutral spine position as the legs lift.
- Squeeze the bottom as you raise the legs to work those buttock muscles a little harder.

ADDITIONAL POSTNATAL EXERCISES

Some selected exercises from the rest of the book to complement your workouts with or without your baby.

Chapter 2: Toning & Strengthening

Swimming (page 56)
Tricep dips (page 60)
Wall squats (page 62)
Prone bottom squeezes (page 65)
Side lying abductor lifts (page 66)
Side lying adductor lifts (page 67)
Trunk curls (page 72)
Ball plank (page 80)
Pelvic lifts (page 81)
Flies (page 87)
Front raises (page 88)
Bicep curls (page 89)

Chapter 3: Aerobics

You can now have a go at the routine in the aerobics section, making sure you just work to your own level and build up duration and intensity gradually. Adapt the routine if necessary, avoiding any exercises that feel uncomfortable.

Chapter 4: Pilates

Side bend (page 135)
The saw (page 136)
Hip rotations (page 139)
Spine curls (page 140)
Kneeling opposite arm and leg extensions (page 146)
Footwork (page 148)
One leg circle (page 150)

Chapter 5: Yoga

Sun salutation (page 164)
Chair pose (page 170)
Warrior 1 (page 173)
Warrior 2 (page 174)
Fan posture (page 179)
Tree pose (page 180)
Crow pose (page 182)
The cat (page 183)
Downward dog (page 185)
Cobra (page 187)
Side plank (page 189)

Chapter 6: Ball Stretches

Ball side bend (page 198)
Standing back stretch (page 200)
Laying chest stretch (page 203)
Spine twist (page 204)
Seated hamstring stretch (page 205)
Front lying quad stretch (page 209)
Frog stretch (page 210)
Ball hug (page 214)

Chapter 9: De-stress

Counting meditation (page 273)
Kneeling torso massage (page 278)
Upper back/neck massage (page 280)
Back rolls (page 283)

HOW LONG AM I POSTNATAL?

This can vary from woman to woman as it is really about how you are feeling. The important consideration is whether the pregnancy hormone relaxin has left your system. Some experts say this can take approximately five months although some believe it may take longer, and isn't until you have stopped breast-feeding. I would suggest that you take into account your pre-pregnancy fitness level and would advise you to listen to your body. When you feel you are ready to move on to more strenuous exercises, you can always consult the book again.

DE-STRESS WITH THE BALL

MEDITATION

People come to meditation for all kinds of reasons and with different expectations. You should approach it as another element of your daily fitness routine and take from it whatever you need, be it stress relief, improved physical or mental health, or a sustained sense of well-being.

You may think of meditation as people sitting around on the floor with their legs crossed, making a rather strange humming sound and generally not doing very much at all. But actually meditation is mental exercise for the mind, in the same way as we have physical exercise for our body. You will be very surprised to find out how hard it is to 'just sit' while meditating. You will want to fidget, phone a friend, make a coffee, turn the television on, anything to avoid just being, but if you can stop worrying about getting things done and allow any thoughts that enter your mind to just pass straight through, then you too will enjoy the power of meditation. Meditation is a buffer zone between you and the stresses of everyday life, an oasis of tranquillity. It will change you by making you more immune to stress, calmer, healthier and filled to the brim with joy.

Using the ball during meditation has lots of added benefits. First, as it is comfortable, it allows us to relax fully into a position without the distraction of an aching back or uncomfortable floor. It is a comforter and allows us the pleasure of touch – like a child with their comfort blanket

or favourite soft toy. The ball can also help us focus on the breath, actually rising and falling if we rest it on our abdomen, ensuring we direct our breath correctly and being a visual clue for our rate of respiration. Throughout this book the ball has become a very dear friend and what could be better than spending more time together.

In this chapter we are going to try just a few of the many different meditation techniques and traditions. They all have one thing in common in that they try to teach you how not to think or how to slow down your thoughts. They use a focusing of attention so that your thoughts are no longer scattered or undirected. It doesn't mean that you are unconscious – you are just trying to let go of the thousands of details that pass frenziedly through the mind. No one can deny that thinking is necessary to us as human beings. The problem is that when we do want to relax for a while, we just keep on thinking. Meditation is about boosting your concentration and focusing your thoughts.
It gives you some time for yourself and puts you in tune with the universe.

BENEFITS OF MEDITATION

- Lowers stress hormones in the blood.
- Reduces cholesterol levels.
- Reduces chances of depression or anxiety.
- Increases confidence.

- Reduces cases of heart disease.
- Clears the mind and creates a calmer state.
- Can help to heal or manage chronic pain.
- Promotes a general feeling of well-being.

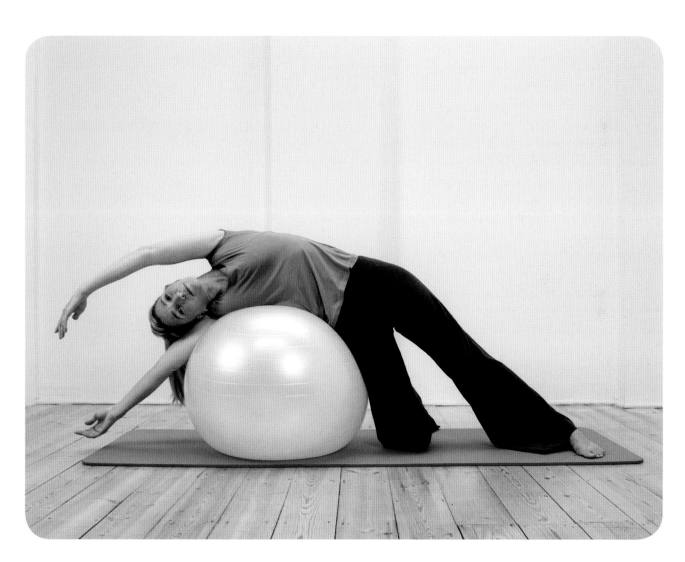

BALL MEDITATION EXERCISES

Before you start the following meditation exercises, make sure you are wearing appropriate clothing to keep you warm and comfortable. Make sure that you will not be disturbed by anyone – turn off your mobile phone and unplug the landline.

SEATED CANDLE MEDITATION

Sit on your ball to start and place a lit candle so that it is at eye level. Make sure you are comfortable and relaxed through your head, neck, shoulders and arms.

Start by bringing your attention to your breath and imagining that each time you exhale you release any remaining tension, until you feel the muscles relax. Now bring your focus to the light of the candle. Steady your mind and clear it of any thoughts. Draw yourself into the light of the flame, feeling the heat wrapping around you as your body melts into the relaxation. If thoughts come into your mind, just let them pass straight through and keep your focus on the candle. Lose yourself in the moving flame and allow your body to relax.

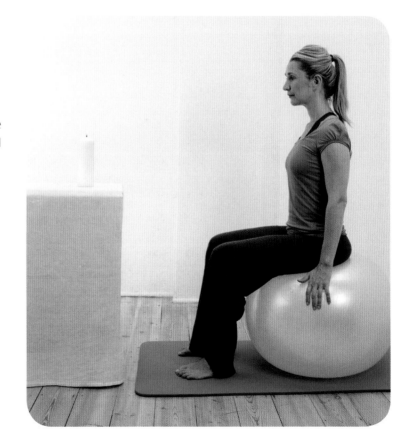

COUNTING MEDITATION

Lie on your back with your ball placed on your abdomen. Check you are comfortable with no areas of tension in the body. Try and keep your arms fully relaxed even though they are keeping the ball in place. Bring your attention now to your breath. Feel the rise and the fall of the ball with each inhalation and exhalation. Become aware of where your breath travels as it comes in through your nose, down into your lungs and then out again through your mouth.

   Bring your focus back to each breath. Using a silent count, inhale for the count of one, then exhale, saying the number one to yourself. Next time you breathe in, say the number two. Count two again as you release the breath. Inhale and count three. Exhale as you count three again. Keep this going until you have reached up to a count of ten and then work back down again. Keep using the same silent count in your head and keep an awareness of the rise and fall of the ball with each breath. If a thought comes into your mind, just let it pass through and return your focus to your silent count. Let the air and the flow release any tension from within the body. When you arrive back to the count of one, bring your focus back to your body. Become aware of how you are feeling.

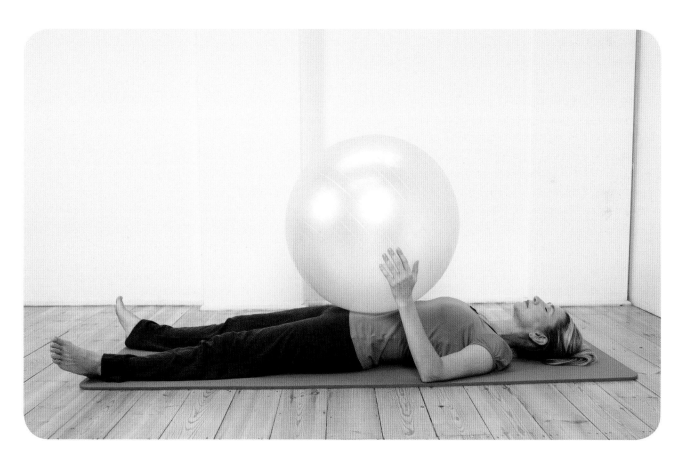

MIND BODY SCAN

Start in the Corpse Pose (see page 193), lying on your back with your feet up on the ball. This is one of the most important yoga postures, as it is designed to bring the body into total conscious relaxation. This pose is easily recreated with the ball and is great for anyone with lower back pain, as it takes pressure away from the lower back while in position. Make sure you feel relaxed and comfortable before you start and that you are not holding any tension in the body.

1 First bring your awareness to your right foot, tense it for a few seconds and then relax it, imagining that it feels very heavy and warm.

2 Now working up your right leg, tense your calf muscle for a few seconds and then release, letting all of the tension flow out of your leg, imagining it to feel heavy and warm.

3 Tense the thigh muscle, release again after a few seconds and allow all of the tension to drift away through the foot, leaving the leg feeling heavy, relaxed and warm. Notice the difference between how your left and right legs feel now.

4 You are now going to repeat with the left leg; notice afterwards if both legs now feel equal.

5 Now squeeze your buttocks tightly for a few seconds and then release, feeling the tension flow away leaving a feeling of heaviness and warmth.

6 Next contract your abdominals for a few seconds; once again relax and release the tension.

7 Now the spine: visualise the tension here, and then imagine it all emptying away through the tailbone, leaving each vertebra feeling heavy and sinking into the floor.

8 Next contract your chest muscles as tightly as you can for a few seconds, and allow all the tension to seep away down the spine and out through the tailbone.

9 Next bring your attention to your left shoulder, tense it tightly so that it comes away from the floor, then allow it to relax and imagine all the tension drifting away through the fingertips.

10 Now tense the rest of your left arm, again relaxing after a few seconds and feeling the tension seep away through the fingertips.

11 And now clench your left fist as tightly as possible, then relax, letting all of the negative energy flow out though your fingertips. Notice now whether your left arm feels different to your right?

12 And now repeat on the right arm, starting from your shoulder; notice again at the end if both arms now feel equal.

13 Now pull your chin back, creating tension in your neck. After a few seconds release and allow any negative energy to flow down your spine and out through your tailbone.

14 Lastly, clench your jaw and screw up your whole face. Then relax the face, imagining the skin and muscles falling towards the back of your head.

15 Now imagine a warm glow of golden light. It begins at your toes and slowly moves up your body to the crown of your head, checking for any tension along the way. If any tense areas are found, allow the light to warm and relax the area.

16 You should now be feeling completely relaxed. Imagine that your body is melting into the ground, your feet melting into the ball. Remain in this position for at least 10 minutes. Stay aware of your breath, breathing deeply, filling the whole body.

17 Now gradually bring your awareness back to your body and your environment. Slowly sit yourself up when you are ready.

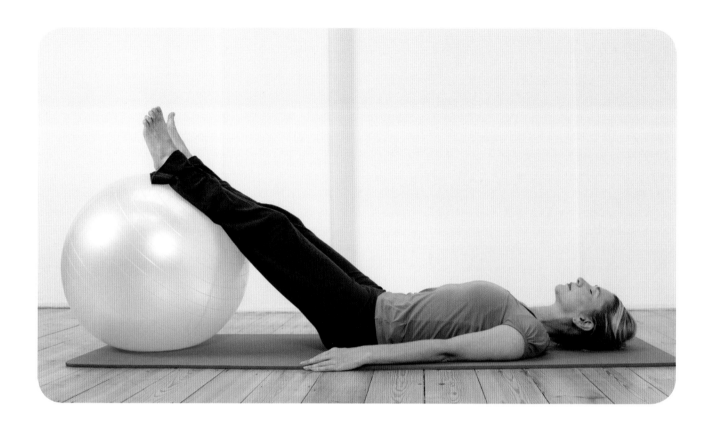

MINDFUL THINKING

Mindfulness is one of the simplest meditation techniques, and yet potentially the most revealing as it involves letting go any desire to control your thoughts, and at the same time not allowing them to control you. At random moments throughout your day, stop what you are doing and consider whether you are in a mindful state of awareness. Are you relaxed and paying attention to the task at hand? Or are you allowing thoughts of what you have to do next, or what you should have done yesterday, distract you? In our efforts for a more productive and efficient lifestyle, we omit something very important – the life part. Learn to live in the present moment and take time to notice.

Try this simple exercise in mindfulness, set a timer for one minute and look out of the window, either at the office or at home. When the timer goes off, write down everything that you have observed in that minute. You can try the same exercise recording only sounds if you like. The more you do this, the longer your list will get, as you become practised at watching mindfully, living in the present moment and taking notice.

BALL SELF-MASSAGE

Massage can both stimulate and relax the body and mind. As tense muscles relax, stiff joints are loosened and nerves soothed, which brings about a general sense of relaxation and well-being. Massage is a very powerful tool. Everyone enjoys massage, from babies to the elderly, from sports men and women to lovers and friends. Every single one of us can benefit in some way from this powerful form of touch.

Using your ball to replace a person in the giving of the massage may seem slightly odd, but some people would prefer not to have such intimate contact with a masseuse and feel much more comfortable with this approach. For those of you who really do enjoy human contact, this isn't to replace those sessions, but is an opportunity for you to self-massage. There are many self-massage products on the market, such as wooden rollers and balls, but there is something about the exercise ball, its shape, texture and gentle touch, that lends itself very well to being the perfect massage partner.

In recent years we are rediscovering the healing powers of massage and other touch therapies, which have been used in other cultures for thousands of years. Massage is becoming more widely acknowledged for its benefits and healing abilities, not only in holistic circles but also throughout the medical profession. While you are restricted with the type of massage strokes you can experience with the ball, it should still be relaxing and serene and should leave your body feeling balanced and revitalised.

KNEELING SHOULDER MASSAGE

? **WHAT FOR?** To release tension in the fronts of the shoulders.

1 **a** Start kneeling with the ball placed underneath the front of your right shoulder and your left hand on the floor for support.

2 **b** Start to draw circles with your right shoulder, pushing it into the ball, trying to cover the whole shoulder area with pressure from the ball.

3 Take 10–15 circles, then repeat on the left side.

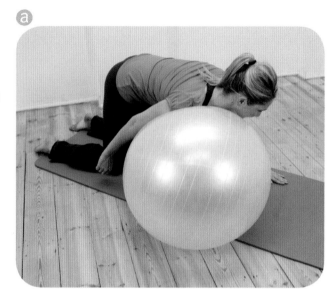

TIPS

- Adjust the pressure against the ball to your own requirements. Some people like their massage to be firm, others prefer it lighter.
- Try and manipulate the whole of the front of the shoulder area with the pressure from the ball. Pay particular attention to any areas that feel tight or tense.

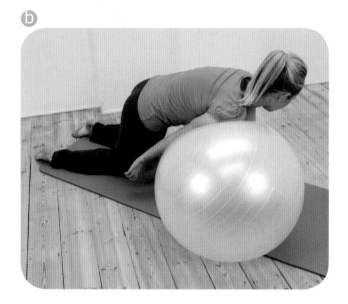

KNEELING TORSO MASSAGE

? WHAT FOR? To release tension from the front of your torso, including the pectoral muscles in the chest and the upper abdominals.

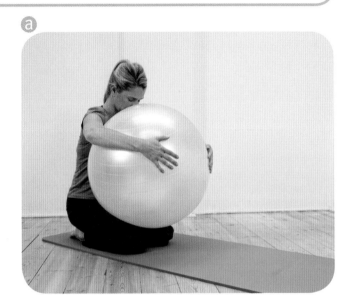

1 **a** Start kneeling with the ball placed on your knees and your arms hugging it.

2 **b** Roll your body forwards allowing the ball to roll off your knees. Keep rolling forwards until the ball rolls as far as your abdominals.

3 Now roll back to your starting position.

4 Repeat the rolls 8–10 times.

TIPS

- Keep a slow, constant pace throughout the rolls, really working through any areas of tension.
- Keep the ball hugged in close to your body.
- It might benefit your relaxation to close your eyes and try and fully relax into the movement.

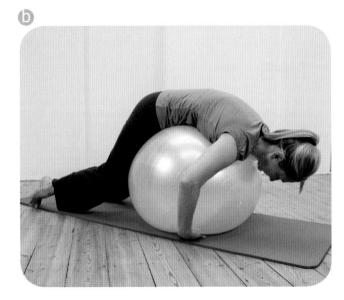

QUADRICEPS MASSAGE

? WHAT FOR? To release any tension from the large muscle in the front of the thighs.

1 **a** Start over the ball with your hands on the floor, the ball underneath your right hip and the ball of your left foot resting on the floor.

2 **b** Use your left foot to initiate the movement. Move so that the ball rolls up your right leg until it is just above your knee and then roll the ball back to your hip. Try making the movement circular so that you travel up one side of the leg and back down the other.

3 Repeat the movement 10–15 times and then repeat on the other leg.

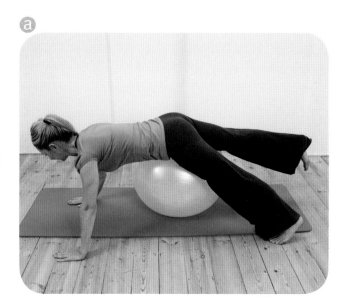

TIPS

- Keep your weight between your two hands and your supporting foot and move your body as far as you need to manipulate the length of the thigh.
- Keep your abdominals engaged throughout the movement to avoid unnecessary pressure on the lower back.

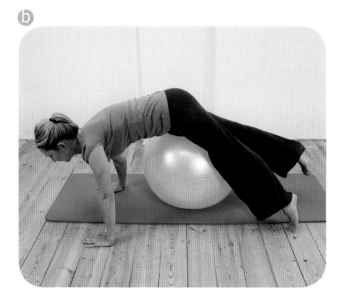

UPPER BACK/NECK MASSAGE

1 **a** Start sitting with your knees bent up and the ball on the floor behind you. Lean back onto the ball so that it is resting underneath your neck and reach your arms overhead to hold the ball in place.

2 **b** Lift your bottom a few inches away from the floor, and then move your body from side to side so the ball rolls first under your right shoulder, then all the way back until it is underneath your left shoulder.

3 Roll from side to side 10–12 times.

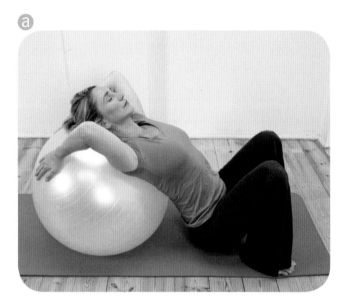

TIPS

- Try to manoeuvre the ball so that it gets into any spots that feel particularly tense.
- Keep a steady pace as you move from side to side, finding your own rhythm to the movement.

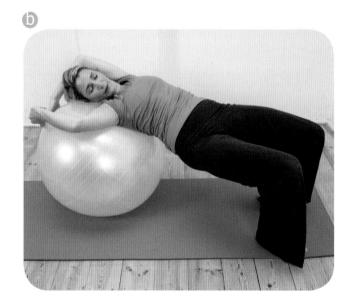

BUTTOCKS MASSAGE

? WHAT FOR? To release any tension from the buttocks and the top of the hamstrings.

1 **ⓐ** Start seated on the ball with your hands resting lightly on your knees or by your sides.

2 **ⓑ** Start to draw large circles with the hips, first to the right making sure that the ball travels across the whole area really manipulating the large muscles in your buttocks.

3 Take 10–15 circles. Repeat to the left side.

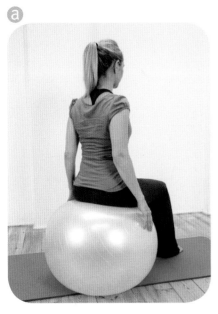

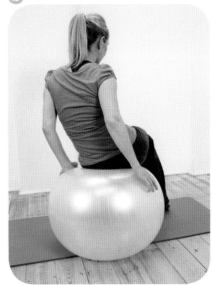

TIP

- Shift your weight around the ball as much as necessary to ensure that the whole buttocks area gets massaged.

SIDE MASSAGE

1 **ⓐ** Start on your knees with the ball by your right side.

2 **ⓑ** Drape your body sideways over the ball, reaching your right arm towards the floor. Reach your left arm overhead and extend your left leg out to the side.

3 Draw circles with the ball over the right side of your body, using your left leg to steer the ball to the areas you would like to massage.

4 Take 10–15 circles. Repeat on the other side.

TIP

- If you lift your chest towards the ceiling, you can work on the back of the shoulder blades too. If you drop the chest towards the floor you target the chest and the ribcage.

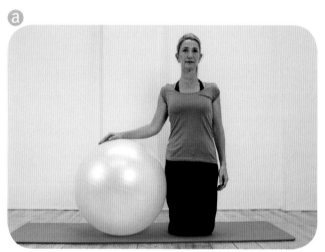

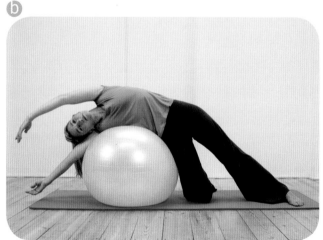

BACK ROLLS

? WHAT FOR? To release tension either side of the spine.

1   Start seated on your ball. Walk yourself out, allowing the ball to roll up your spine, **a** stopping when it is underneath your shoulder blades. **b** Make sure the ball is not resting on the spine – you should feel it on the muscles to the side of the vertebrae.

2   **c** Place your left hand behind your head, supporting the neck, and move your weight so that the ball is resting on the right hand side of the back.

3   **d** Straighten your legs allowing the ball to roll all the way down to your lower back.

4   **e** Bend your knees allowing the ball to roll all the way up to the neck.

5   Keep rolling the ball up and down the right side of the back 10–15 times. Repeat on the left side.

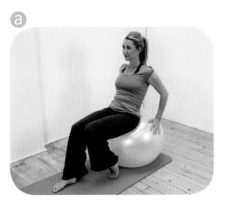

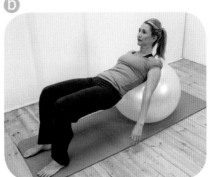

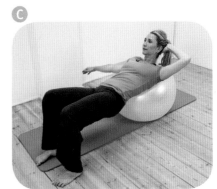

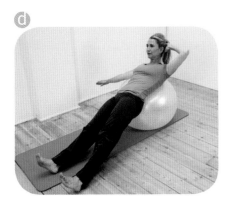

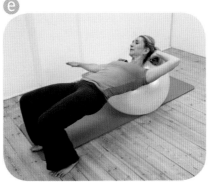

TIPS

- Keep your neck relaxed into the supporting hand.
- Keep the movement steady, slowing down and working out any areas of tension.

RESOURCES

www.physicalcompany.co.uk
The Physical Company
01494 769222
Sells balls, pumps, ball carry straps, mats and other exercise equipment.

www.fitballs.co.uk
Proactive Health
0800 434 6170
Everything to do with balls.

www.halfords.com
Halfords
They sell a great electric pump that plugs into your car lighter and inflates the ball in no time at all.

www.yoga.com
Everything to do with yoga, including a wide range of products to buy, articles to read and forums for discussion.

www.pilates.co.uk
Everything about Pilates, including a class finder and a shop for all those essentials.

www.meditationexpert.co.uk
Everything about meditation, including various techniques and an option for you to ask an expert a question.

www.nct.org.uk
National Childbirth Trust
Lots of information about pregnancy, birthing and becoming a parent, including exercise advice.

www.imcvision.com
IMC Vision
01923 718800
On this website you can purchase any of my gymball, Pilates and general fitness DVDs. There is also an extensive range of other good-quality healthy living/fitness programmes available to buy. Definitely worth a look.

www.balldynamics.com
Ball Dynamics International
US-based international suppliers of the ball.

www.knowyourbodybest.com
1-800-881-1681
Know Your Body Best
Canadian distributor of exercise balls and other exercise equipment.

INDEX

A

abdominal bracing **256**
abdominal exercises **72–79**
abdominal separation **257**
acclimatisation **15**
adductor squeezes **69, 264**
aerobics **94–125**
  benefits **97**
  complete routine **122–125**
  getting started **97**
antenatal exercises **242–249**
arm circles **137**

B

baby chest press **259**
baby curl ups **261**
baby, exercises with **258–265**
back extensions on the ball **224**
back rolls **283**
back rowing **142–143**
ball balance **147**
ball benefits **8–9**
ball front raises **54**
ball hugs **214**
ball plank **80**
ball reaches **233**
ball rolls **157**
ball side bend **198**
ball size guide **12**
ball spine curls **213**
ball squats **64**
ball stretches **194–217**
base positions **20–23**
bicep curls **89**

birthing with the ball **250–253**
boat pose **186**
body mechanics **236**
bouncing on the ball **33**
bow pose **191**
breathing **24**
  breathing with arm raises **163**
  diaphragmatic breathing exercise **162**
  exercises **25–27**
  Pilates **131**
  yoga **161**
bridge balance **227**
buttocks massage **281**

C

Caesarean delivery **254**
calf raises **263**
candle pose **188**
cat, the **183**
chair pose **170–171**
chest lifts **232**
chest openings **234**
chest press **86**
chest stretch **235**
cobra **187**
complete routines
  warm up **48–49**
  aerobics **122–125**
core muscles, engaging **19**
corpse pose **193**
counting meditation **273**
crow pose **182**

D

de-stress with the ball **268–283**
donkey jumps with ball bounce **119**
double leg cycles **78**
double leg lifts **93**
double leg stretch **154**
double side steps **109**
downward dog **185**

E

engaging the core **19**
exercise balls **6**
  benefits **8–9**
  care **13**
  choosing **12**
  equipment **14**
  inflating **12**
  space required **13**
exercises (to tone & strengthen) **52**
  abdominal **72–79**
  full body integration **80–83**
  lower body **62–71**
  upper body **54–61**
  using hand weights **84–93**

F

fan posture **179**
figure of 8 arm circles **40**
flies **87**
foot taps **36**
footwork **148–149**
forward baby raises **258**
forward bend with wide legs **245**
forward fold **169**

four-step turn **114–115**
frog stretch **210**
front lying quad stretch **209**
front raises **88**
full body integration **80–83**
full body stretch **216–217**

G
getting started **10–49**
grapevines **112–13**

H
half jacks **35**
half stand ups **38**
hamstring curls **70–71, 117**
hand weights **14, 52, 84**
    exercises using **86–93**
    making your own **84**
healthy back and posture **218–237**
hedgehog, the **144**
hip and bottom stretch **207**
hip circles **30**
hip rotations **139**
hoover **55**
hundred, the **141**

I
incline position **20**

J
jacks **102**
jump squats **116**
jumping knee lifts **120**

K
knee lifts with ball roll **134**
kneeling balance **82–83**
kneeling ball rolls **79**
kneeling cat stretch **243**

kneeling chest stretch **202**
kneeling forward with ball support **251**
kneeling inner thigh stretch **208**
kneeling opposite arm and leg extensions **146**
kneeling shoulder massage **277**
kneeling torso massage **278**

L
lat pull downs against wall **228**
leg beats **68**
lifting **236**
look right and left **29**
lower body exercises **62–71**
lunge stretch **206**
lunge with ball support **47**
lunges with arms **104–105**
lying back extensions **225**
lying chest stretch **203**
lying double arm rows **91**
lying hamstring stretch **212**

M
marching with ball punches **110**
massage **276–283**
meditation **270**
    ball meditation exercises **272–275**
    benefits **271**
mind body scan **274**
mindful thinking **275**
mobility **230–235**
mountain pose **166**

N
neck massage **280**
neutral spine **16**
    seated neutral position **18**
    standing neutral position **17**

O
oblique curls against the wall **74**
oblique twists **92**
one leg balance **167**
one leg circle **150–151**
opposite arm and leg raises **226**

P
peek-a-boo rows **260**
pelvic circles **244**
pelvic floor **255**
    pelvic floor exercises **247**
pelvic lifts **81**
pelvic tilts **132**
Pilates **126–157**
    breathing practice **131**
    eight principles **130**
    exercises **132–157**
    what is **128**
Pilates, Joseph **129**
pose of the child **192**
pose of the dancer **176**
postnatal exercises **254–256**
posture **220–223**
    good body mechanics **236**
    lying **223**
    mobility exercises **230–235**
    sitting **222**
    standing **221**
    strengthening exercises **224–229**
pregnancy, birthing and beyond **238–267**
    antenatal exercises **242–249**
    benefits of exercise **241**
    birthing exercises **250–253**
    exercises with baby **258–265**
    post six-week check **257**
    postnatal exercises **254–256**
    pre six-week check **254**

safety **241**
press ups **58–59**
   against the wall **246**
prone bottom squeezes **65**
prone position **23**
pyramid pose **172**

Q
quad stretch **46**
quadriceps massage **279**

R
rear leg raises with a raspberry! **265**
resistance training **52**
reverse plank **190**
rock and squat **262**
rocks from side to side **37, 101**
roll up, the **155**
rollover, the **156**
rotating curls **231**
running and bouncing **111**

S
salsa jumps **118**
saw, the **136**
scissor leg reverse curls **75**
seated arm circles **31**
seated ball balance **229**
seated base position **20**
seated bounces **98**
seated candle meditation **272**
seated curl downs **230**
seated hamstring stretch **41, 205**
seated inner thigh stretch **211**
seated one-leg extensions **34**
seated side reaches **32**
seated tricep stretch **201**
seated walking **20**
self-massage **276**

exercises **277–83**
short spine preparation **152**
shoulder isolations **138**
shoulder stretch **44**
side bend **135, 168**
side lying abductor lifts **66**
side lying adductor lifts **67**
side lying oblique curls **76–77**
side lying position **22**
side lying side stretch **215**
side massage **282**
side plank **189**
side-to-side ball rocks **242**
single leg stretch **153**
single side steps **108**
sitting at a computer **236**
spine curls **140**
spine twist **133, 204**
squats **39**
squatting against the ball **252**
stand up sit downs **100**
standing arm lifts **103**
standing back stretch **200**
standing cat stretch **199**
standing foot taps with chest press
   arms **42–43**
standing jobs **236**
standing lean **253**
step touch **99**
stretches **196**
   developmental stretches **196**
   dynamic stretches **197**
   full body stretches **213–217**
   lower body stretches **205–212**
   older people **197**
   static stretches **196**
   upper body stretches **198–204**
sun salutation **164–165**
supine position **21**

swan dive, the **145**
swimming **56–57**
swings side to side **107**

T
temple pose **178**
thread the needle **184**
toning and strengthening **50–93**
tree pose **180–181**
tricep dips **60–61**
tricep extensions **90**
tricep stretch **45**
trunk curls **72–73**

U
upper back/neck massage **280**
upper body exercises **54–61**

W
walking plank **121**
walks around the ball **106**
wall squats **62–63**
warming up **28**
   warm up exercises **29–47**
   warm up routine **48–49**
warrior 1 **173**
warrior 2 **174–5**
warrior 3 **177**
weights **84–93**
wide leg seated position **250**

Y
yoga **158–193**
   breath **161–163**
   postures on and under the ball
      178–191
   relaxation postures **192–193**
   standing postures **166–177**
   sun salutation **164–165**

AUTHOR'S ACKNOWLEDGEMENTS

For my son, Finn, an addition to my life since I last wrote, who has given me so much sunshine and happiness over the last 4 years – it has changed my life forever! Such an affectionate and gorgeous little man, he makes me very proud and fills my heart with love.

For my friend Karen, tragically killed whilst helping people in need of medical care in a remote area of Afghanistan. May her legacy live on and her bravery and compassion inspire others. To help support the continuation of her work visit www.karenwoofoundation.org

And for my partner Ken and my family for continuing to support me through the twists and turns of life.

Thanks also to my publisher Kyle Cathie for continuing to support my work, my editor Catharine Robertson, photographer Tony Chau and designer Heidi Baker.